T0366946

Global Politics of Health

GLOBAL POLITICS OF HEALTH

SARA E. DAVIES

polity

First published in 2009 by Polity Press

Polity Press
65 Bridge Street
Cambridge CB2 1UR, UK

Polity Press
350 Main Street
Malden, MA 02148, USA

ISBN-13: 978-0-7456-4042-6
ISBN-13: 978-0-7456-4041-9(pb)

A catalogue record for this book is available from the British Library.

Typeset in 10.5 on 12 pt Times
by Toppan Best-set Premedia Limited
Printed and bound in Great Britain by MPG Books Limted, Bodmin, Cornwall

The publisher has used its best endeavours to ensure that the URLs for external websites referred to in this book are correct and active at the time of going to press. However, the publisher has no responsibility for the websites and can make no guarantee that a site will remain live or that the content is or will remain appropriate.

Every effort has been made to trace all copyright holders, but if any have been inadvertently overlooked the publisher will be pleased to include any necessary credits in any subsequent reprint or edition.

For further information on Polity, visit our website: www.politybooks.com

CONTENTS

Dedication

I dedicate this book to my darling husband, Alex
– my source of eternal light

ACKNOWLEDGEMENTS

There are many who deserve my gratitude for their assistance over the duration of this book's development and completion. First, I must thank my editor at Polity Press, Louise Knight, and associate editors Rachel Donnelly and Emma Hutchinson. Thank you for your encouragement, engagement and patience – I could not have completed this book without your support.

I would like to thank the School of Justice and Faculty of Law at Queensland University of Technology for being so supportive at the beginning of this journey. A big thank you to Zoe Staines, who faithfully worked as my research assistant for six months. My recent home, the Centre for Governance and Public Policy and Griffith Asia Institute at Griffith University, has been a wonderful place to complete the book. The support from all the staff, especially Jason Sharman, Patrick Weller and Michael Wesley, has meant that I was able to finish the book in peace but with the knowledge that I could always find encouragement in the corridors if required. I would also like to especially thank colleagues who have inspired and generously assisted me along this journey: Roland Bleiker, Melissa Curley, Christian Enemark, Yasmin Grey, Caroline Hyde-Price, Kelly Lee, Colin McInnes, Simon Rushton and Barbara Sullivan. Writing a book that seeks to incorporate two distinct disciplines means that I will have made a lot of mistakes and all, of course, are my own. Thank you to those who read and commented on the manuscript, including the two anonymous reviewers. Their detailed comments and insights have, I hope, improved the book.

Finally, I would like to thank my brilliant, loving and generous family. My parents, Marie and Alan – thank you for your belief and encouragement, strength and love. My sisters, Jane and Clair – thank you for being not just sisters, but my best friends. My brothers-in-law, Tony and James, thank you for your constant love, support and patience.

It is fitting that a very special and cherished family member, our little child, arrived before the completion of this book. Words cannot express how much you mean to me, Isaac. I will endeavour to always provide you with the means to health and happiness, and make you proud. I love you to the moon and back.

Last, but never least, thank you my darling husband, Alex. This book exists only because of your patience, love, dedication and kindness. The best I am and have is because of you. I cherish you and will love you always.

Sara Davies, Brisbane, 2009

ABBREVIATIONS

AMC	Advanced Market Commitment
AIDS	Acquired Immune Deficiency Syndrome
ARVs	Antiretrovirals
CEDAW	Convention against the Elimination of Discrimination Against Women
CL	Compulsory Licensing
CRO	Contract Research Organization
CROC	Convention on the Rights of the Child
CSDH	Commission on Social Determinants of Health
DALYs	DisabilityAdjusted Life Years
DRC	Democratic Republic of Congo
DTP3	Diphtheria, Tetanus and Pertussis vaccination
EID(s)	Emerging Infectious Disease(s)
EU	European Union
FAO	Food and Agriculture Organization
G8	Group of Eight States
GATT	General Agreement on Tariff and Trade
GATS	General Agreement on Trade in Services
GAVI	Global Alliance for Vaccines and Immunization
GDP	Gross Domestic Product
GNP	Gross National Product
GOARN	Global Outbreak Alert Response Network
GPA	Global Program on AIDS
GPEI	Global Polio Eradication Initiative
GPHIN	Global Health Information Network
H5N1	Strain of Avian Influenza

HIV	Human Immunodeficiency Virus
ICC	International Criminal Court
ICESCR	International Covenant on Economic, Social and Cultural Rights
ICPD	International Conference on Population and Development
ICRC	International Committee of the Red Cross
IDP(s)	Internally Displaced Person(s)
IHR	International Health Regulations
ILO	International Labour Organization
IMF	International Monetary Fund
IPEH	International Political Economy of Health
IR	International Relations (discipline of)
IRC	International Rescue Committee
MDGs	Millennium Development Goals
MSF	Médecins Sans Frontières
NGO(s)	Non-Governmental Organization(s)
OCHA	Office for the Coordination of Humanitarian Affairs
OECD	Organization for Economic Cooperation and Development
OIE	World Organization for Animal Health
PHEIC	Public Health Emergency of International Concern
PI	Parallel Importing
PPP	Public–Private Partnership
ProMED Mail	Program for Monitoring Emerging Diseases
PRSP	Poverty Reduction Strategy Papers
PYLL	Potential Years of Life Lost
QALYs	Quality-Adjusted Life Years
REID(s)	Re-Emerging Infectious Diseases
SARS	Severe Acute Respiratory Syndrome
SAPs	Structural Adjustment Programs
SHOC	Strategy Health Operations Centre
STD(s)	Sexually Transmitted Disease(s)
TB	Tuberculosis
TRIPS	Trade-Related aspects of Intellectual Property Rights
UN	United Nations
UNESCO	United Nations Educational, Scientific and Cultural Organization
UNGA	United Nations General Assembly
UNODC	United Nations Office of Drugs and Crime
UNSC	United Nations Security Council
UNAIDS	Joint United Nations Programme on HIV/AIDS

UNDP	United Nations Development Programme
UNFPA	United Nations Population Fund
UNHCR	United Nations High Commissioner for Refugees
UNICEF	United Nations Children's Emergency Fund
USAID	United States Agency for International Development
US CDC	United States Centers for Disease Control
US DoD	United States Department of Defense
WHA	World Health Assembly
WHO	World Health Organization
WTO	World Trade Organization

INTRODUCTION

I first started work on this book shortly after the end of the SARS crisis in 2003 and the initial H5N1 avian influenza outbreak in Vietnam, Indonesia, Thailand and China. I thought that those concerned with world politics needed to understand that health is a political issue that impacts at the local, national and global levels. Good health and the opportunity to seek health care are of intrinsic value for making progress in international relations between states and between conflicting groups within states. Furthermore, the actors that assume a role in establishing the conditions for good health and health care are no longer exclusively local and national governments. An increasing number of non-state actors such as the Bill and Melinda Gates Foundation are funding local health projects, and international organizations such as the World Health Organization and World Bank contribute to, and shape domestic and global health policy.

The aim of this book is threefold. First, to demonstrate the need for International Relations (IR) scholars to study public health issues in the same manner that peacekeeping, global governance and defence arrangements are studied. Second, to highlight issues deserving more attention and deliberation. Third, to propose directions for further study.

Traditionally, public health policy embodied the study of the interaction of people and patterns of disease (Lakoff 2008: 38–39). From its origins in nineteenth-century Britain, the study of public health focused almost exclusively on domestic issues. The field's relatively short history has led scholars of IR to forget – as Andrew Price-Smith (2009) recently demonstrated – that health has a long history as a core component of 'high politics'. In this book, I define 'high politics' as political matters related to the state's survival (Booth 1996: 337; Buzan et al. 1998a: 388–390).[1] But not until the recent emergence of high-profile infectious diseases such as SARS and HIV, has health been seen once again as a concern for those shaping foreign policy. IR has therefore traditionally neglected an empirically rich area of relations between states, and between states and other actors. As a result, the discipline has missed the link between health and issues central to world politics such as globalization, human rights, war, humanitarian emergencies, economics and development, and international law.

The thirty countries of the Organization for Economic Co-operation and Development (OECD) are home to less than 20% of the world's population but their spending on health is 90% of the world's total health expenditure (WHO 2007a: 19). According to one estimate, if US$66 billion was invested in low-income countries to address essential health needs, by 2015/2020 such an investment could generate economic benefits of $360 billion per year (Sachs 2002: 1; WHO 2002: 12–13). Globally, women and children are at higher risk from malnutrition, violence, sexually transmitted diseases (STDs) and respiratory illness due to their weak political, economic and social position; while the elderly and disabled often account for high numbers of internally displaced persons (IDPs). This makes them just as vulnerable as children to malnutrition and poor health (MSF 1997: 27; Salama et al. 2001: 1430). Women bear the brunt of global health inequalities. For example, in 2007 women accounted for 61% of HIV infections in sub-Saharan Africa. In Latin America, Asia and Eastern Europe the proportion of women becoming HIV infected is increasing (UNAIDS 2007). Likewise, between 1990 and 2005, while there was an overall decrease of 2.5% per year in the maternal mortality ratio, there were still 535,900 maternal deaths in 2005 and the ratios in sub-Saharan Africa showed little if any improvement (Hill et al. 2007).

Each day, 4,500 children die from *preventable* diseases (WHO 2007b: 4).[2] The life expectancy of a child born in Afghanistan is 42, while in Sweden it is 81 (WHO 2008a: 36, 42). Malaria, tuberculosis (TB) and HIV/AIDS still account for one-third of all deaths due to infectious disease, but the majority of deaths caused by infectious disease are from diarrhoeal disease and respiratory infections (UN 2007). To make matters worse, between 2002 and 2007, forty new diseases emerged and there were 1,100 reported epidemics of infectious disease (WHO 2007b: x). Sanitation receives less than 0.5% of GDP spending in developing countries – yet basic sanitation could stop at least 40% of diarrhoeal disease in these countries (George 2008).[3] This means that at least half of the children who die today could have been saved by sewage disposal systems.

All of these deaths and suffering are the result (whether directly or indirectly) of local and international political decisions. Good health is vital for good politics and vice versa. Ironically, even war – the stuff of traditional high politics – needs healthy people ready for combat duty. However, students of IR are rarely called on to think about how the provision of health care may be as important a factor for winning a war as armaments and strategies.[4] In short, a comprehensive picture of IR must consider the relationship between health and world politics.

How then might IR attempt to understand this relationship? One approach, which this book develops, is to consider health problems and responses that involve actors both within and outside the state whose behaviour shapes and impacts on health policies, problems and capacities. Moreover, in looking at how public health policy is shaped by a range of different actors, I argue that the conceptualization of particular health issues as matters of either 'high politics' or 'low politics' shapes how they are framed and pursued politically. This, in turn, can impact on long-term health outcomes, though as I point out in chapter 1, it is not always the case that conceptualizing issues as matters of high politics produces more effective health outcomes.

This book, it should be stressed, has some limitations. I do not have medical training and, therefore, my understanding of epidemiology, biomedicine, pharmacy, physiology, psychology and humanitarian work is filtered through discussions with those who do have such backgrounds. I have read widely in medical textbooks and journals, and have done my best to come to grips with a scientific field that has brought about enormous improvements in health, especially in the last 60 years. This book seeks to understand the interconnection between health and world politics. As such, it does not spend much time on the health policies of individual states.

Layout of the book

In chapter 1, I map the way in which IR has engaged with public health and set out a framework that guides the remainder of the book. I identify two key perspectives on the relationship between health and world politics, which, for heuristic purposes, I label 'statist' and 'globalist'. Both perspectives make the case for taking health seriously, but whereas statists' focus is on the state as the primary referent, globalists suggest that individuals should be the referent. The statist perspective uses the language of security to promote particular health issues to the realm of 'high politics'. In contrast, the globalist perspective does not assume that the state is necessarily the most significant or legitimate actor for delivering health to individuals. Instead, this approach takes the individual as its starting point and explores what threatens individuals and how those threats can be addressed. It is not uncommon for both perspectives to converge and borrow from each other in their approach to health issues. For example, some who espouse globalist ambitions have used the language of securitization promoted by the statist perspective to call for more resources to be devoted to global health. Using the prism of statist and globalist perspectives allows us to understand contemporary debates and to identify the underlying issues involved. Chapter 1 identifies a tension within IR regarding the possibility of studying health issues without the need to justify such studies through the language of security, which inevitably narrows the scope of health issues that can be explored and frames the way in which they are studied.

The chapters that follow will demonstrate that a variety of global health issues are underscored by these tensions about the appropriate referent for global health (the state or the individual) and the appropriate source of health remedies (the state or an admixture of states and other types of actor). To date, approaches to the global politics of health have tended to either prioritize the security of the state or the security of the individual. The idea of doing both at the same time is rarely considered. Having outlined the way in which IR tends to think about health and international relations, chapter 2 maps the key actors that are engaged in the global politics of health. The emphasis here is on 'global', not just 'international' actors, reflecting the emergence of state-based and *non-state*-based actors. Key actors include states, traditional international organizations such as WHO and the World Bank, humanitarian non-state actors such as Médecins Sans Frontières (MSF), and philanthropic actors such as the Bill and Melinda Gates Foundation (referred to as the Gates Foundation). These actors have developed differing degrees of influence over health policies and outcomes, and as a result it is becoming harder to identify patterns of influence and the myriad ways in which actors relate to and impact on one another. It is important to recognize though that this complex combination of actors has not led to the state becoming a less significant health actor. Instead, states and various types of non-state actor have established interdependent relationships, raising important dilemmas about the appropriate locus of responsibility for the provision of health care which mirror the tensions identified by the statist and globalist perspectives. These dilemmas reappear in different guises in all the chapters that follow.

Having looked at the main approaches that shape the way that IR views health and identified the principal actors engaged in what has been described as 'global health governance', the remaining chapters focus on specific public health issues that (1) span borders, (2) require interstate co-operation and regulation and (3) have vertical reach – in that a policy or funding decision made by a global actor can affect the health of individuals. Five thematic issues that satisfy these three conditions are the focus of the remainder of the book: health as a human right, cross-border migration, civil and interstate conflict, the prevention of infectious disease, and health goods as a business.

In chapter 3, I evaluate the question of whether health should be understood as a human right, and the impact of doing so. The 'health as a human right' movement, which developed in the 1980s, was a direct response to the fact that health issues were quickly losing political ground at a time when the small progress made in extending life expectancy and reducing child mortality globally was in danger in poorer regions of the world. The rise of HIV infections in the developing world, and the discrimination that followed, propelled figures such as the late Jonathan Mann to argue that public health needed new foundations from which to claim political significance. However, as this chapter will argue by tracing the HIV awareness and reproductive health campaigns, evoking human rights has led to some uneven outcomes. Adherence to the globalist perspective, where the rights and needs of the individual justify the conceptualization of health as a human right, results in a categorical imperative claim at the global political level that is yet to be won. This is largely because there remains uncertainty about what the outcome is meant to look like and what different actors are responsible for in a context where the state remains the primary actor for interpreting and realizing these rights.

Chapter 4 examines how cross-border migration evokes another tension between statist and globalist perspectives. Whether the migrant groups are defined as refugees or economic migrants, their health status can be both a cause for flight and used by others to determine their fate. In the first section of the chapter, I look at the dependence that refugees, especially those in camp settlements, have on health assistance from non-governmental actors and international organizations. I trace how the globalist perspective has prevailed with the broad consensus that international actors have a responsibility to keep refugee populations alive but show that, ultimately, vulnerable populations still need to contend with statist realities – especially the political consequences of asking states to host such populations and providing assistance amid a political and military conflict. Humanitarian medical assistance has become part of the war process and therefore camp populations sometimes become further victimized and manipulated through their need for assistance. This raises the question of whether the proliferation of humanitarian actors allows governments to avoid their responsibility to protect their citizens' right to be safe from harm. This

leads to deep moral and political questions about the unintended consequences of aid. In the second part of chapter 4, I explore the experience
of migrants and refugees in high-income countries, as illegal and legal
entrants. How states respond to both migrants and refugees is shaped
by how these groups are conceptualized. In this regard, statism tends
to dominate the way in which states and societies regard incoming
migrants and refugees – with these groups often seen as either a health
threat to be deterred or an unwelcome health burden. This chapter argues
that the way that the health of migrants and refugees is conceptualized
is often deeply rooted in either globalist or statist perspectives, related
to this deep tension between the rights of the individual and the rights of
the state.

There are few worse environments where political conflict collides
with health outcomes than in situations of war. In chapter 5, I explore how
armed conflict exacerbates the vulnerability of civilians and how questions
about medical treatment in war bring their own political ramifications for
soldiers and aid agencies alike. These health questions are typically left
unexplored in IR's accounts of war.[5] While medical improvements have
allowed soldiers to endure war for longer in the twentieth and twenty-first
centuries, we still have little understanding of how health is linked to the
continuation of war and what impact this relationship has on the prospects
for peace. This chapter traces the impact of health on war, examines how
the dead are counted and why this matters, the treatment of wounded civilians and soldiers in war zones, the concept and practice of humanitarian
neutrality in times of war, and the importance of health to peace-building.
Underlying all this are broader tensions about the competing prioritization
of national security and human security, and the withdrawal of the state
from the provision of public health in the context of state failure or protracted civil war.

In chapter 6, I explore the first of two public health issues that have a
relatively long tradition of being understood as a global political issue.
This chapter examines how efforts to prevent the spread of infectious
disease have achieved the status of 'high politics' through being framed
in the language of threat and security. Emphasis has recently been placed
on international co-operative agreements to contain and respond to infectious disease outbreaks, and success in this area has been, arguably, largely
due to the focus on threat prevention – particularly among developed states
and the WHO. The impact of this securitized approach to infectious disease
is twofold. On the one hand, greater interest in infectious disease means
greater interest in health at the global level, which can have positive outcomes in terms of increased investment. On the other hand, there is also
the possibility that securitization frames the problem of infectious disease

in a way that could work against populations plagued by communicable disease: where the 'unwell' (poor) are ignored in order to protect the 'well' (rich) from the spread of infectious disease; where diseases that could spread to the global North are prioritized over those – more deadly diseases – that are unlikely to do so. I argue that responses to infectious disease are dominated by statism and securitization, and involve focusing on containing the threat of infectious disease rather than tackling its root causes. Why this has been the most popular response among wealthy governments is obvious, but its capacity to deliver health improvement outcomes for all is less clear.

In the final chapter, I focus on the second area of public health that has already received a significant degree of interest among global actors. The international political economy of health (IPEH) has given us a good understanding of how local, national and international political and economic forces coalesce to determine access to health. In this chapter, I argue that IPEH is shaped by two particular approaches of its own, which I label 'utilitarian' and 'health equity'. Similar to the statist and globalist perspectives, the utilitarian and health equity approaches take opposing views on the key referents. Utilitarians subscribe to the idea that the state should play a stabilizing role in ensuring that health care can be provided to its citizens, but some utilitarians go a step further and argue that at a certain point the state may also have to give way to free market influences. The health equity approach argues that the needs and rights of individuals must be the priority in shaping IPEH, and (even more so than the globalist perspective) calls for the state to play a leading role in ensuring health equity and access.

The chapter unpacks this debate by examining four cases – prescription medicines, clinical offshore trials, vaccination trials and health tourism – tracing the positions taken in each according to my broadly defined utilitarian and health equity perspectives. I argue that the utilitarian position focuses on the role of economic utility in determining what level of health care individuals should have access to, based largely on neoliberal principles of the free market. By contrast, the health equity perspective is based on the view of health as a human right and aims to ensure that health access is *not* determined by neoliberal free market principles because of the inherent inequality that this system produces. In each of these four areas, global actors such as international organizations and multinational corporations influence the level of health access that is available to individuals around the world. I argue that both perspectives in IPEH, as with statist and globalist perspectives more broadly, need to accept that they borrow from each other's positions and thus both contain a degree of truth. While, on the one hand, utilitarians are right to argue that providing the best health care for the greatest number of people has not always been achieved through state-run health systems, on the other hand, health equity advocates are also right to highlight that global non-state actors have even less of a social contract to ensure citizens' well-being and that neoliberalism produces greater health inequality. In sum, with IPEH and IR in general, the relationship between public health and world politics is not a rigid hierarchical one whereby the state impacts on the individual and international co-operative mechanisms impact the state. The relationship is more fluid than this. For example, international trade agreements can dramatically affect an individual's health, sometimes in spite of the state's attempt to block this impact. Likewise, individuals are increasingly seeking health remedies outside their own state, further blurring the relationship between the individual, the state and global health governance.

There are many global health issues yet to receive the sustained level of attention that infectious disease and access to essential medicines have received. The next step is to consider why this must be the case. IR's approach to health tends to focus on the security of either the individual (globalist) or the state (statist). In this book, I argue that the problem is not so much this distinction, but the premise that IR can only contribute to the study and practice of health through the language of security. This narrow focus on security had led us to stop asking why we think more attention on particular health issues brings more security than others in the first place. IR needs to take health seriously, and not just as a means of security, but also in order to better understand the political, economic and social variables that shape health issues and impact on the political relations between states and non-state actors.

1 UNDERSTANDING THE GLOBAL POLITICS OF HEALTH

This chapter examines how the field of International Relations (IR) has come to understand particular public health issues. The international politics of health is best understood according to two principal perspectives: the statist, which is primarily focused on public health as a means through which the stability of the state can be assured, and the globalist, which is primarily focused on securing the well-being and rights of individuals. In this chapter, I will chart both of these perspectives and demonstrate how both have the potential to shape our understanding of the contribution that IR can make to the evolving international health agenda. I outline how these two perspectives frame the current dilemmas that face IR in relation to understanding public health issues. I argue that the field is trapped at present by an impulse to elevate certain public health issues as security concerns when, in fact, security may not be a useful language for describing and institutionalizing effective political responses to particular health problems that affect many individuals around the world.

Health sociologists have long argued that the study of health has been too heavily focused on the individual's relationship with medically defined problems (Turner 1997; Germov 1999; Nettleton 2006). Originally, the study and practice of health was primarily located at the micro level (see figure 1.1) and was concerned with how the medical profession could treat an individual's health problems to produce physiological and psychological wellness. Among other things, this focus excluded the influence of the social environment on an individual's health and, for health sociologists, the health of the individual is determined by the wider social context. They

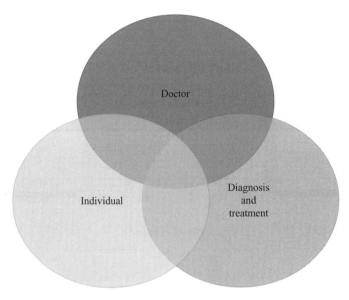

Figure 1.1   Health at the micro level – clinical medicine

maintain that it is only through understanding the scientific as well as economic, cultural and political contexts that shape health that we can identify what being healthy means and how health can best be achieved. In the nineteenth and early twentieth century, doctors typically treated illness as a microcosm, when in fact there was a macrocosm of factors that shaped an individual's health. In other words, it is important to recognize that there is a *macro* context behind the local relationship between a medical practitioner and a patient (Turner 1997; Nettleton 2006). Therefore, good health is best delivered by understanding its micro and macro dimensions (Powles and Comim 2003). While clinical medicine is vital for treating the health of individuals, public health emerged to fill this 'macro' gap and study how the health of the population can be influenced and determined by the social, economic and political context (see figure 1.2).

When we extrapolate upward to the international realm, the number of relevant agents and contexts expands dramatically. National health policies and provisions are intertwined with international considerations about how states relate to each other and to other actors. At the same time, wider international societal norms, politics and economics influence expectations about what can and should be achieved, and how health

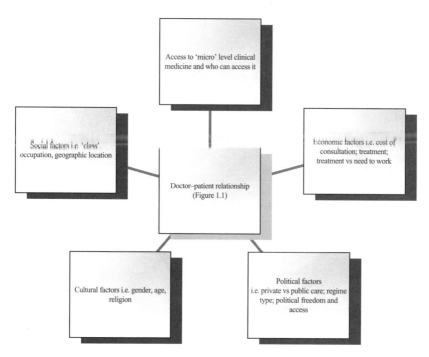

Figure 1.2   Health at the macro level – public health

should be pursued. A range of actors, such as foreign governments, non-governmental organizations (NGOs), pharmaceutical companies, private donors and international organizations, drive a variety of different health agendas that influence priorities within individual states and affect the resources that are available to individual health workers and opportunities for patients. For example, the post-World War II Bretton Woods system had a profound influence on health care policy around the world through the lending practices of institutions such as the World Bank (see chapter 2). As a result, good health is not determined exclusively by an individual's lifestyle, their doctor or local community. The state, the society of states and a range of other actors including international organizations, NGOs and transnational corporations all have the power to shape health opportunities and outcomes. This is where IR can contribute profound insight into how and why these actors have accumulated such power, and how this blurring of the 'domestic' and 'international' realm of health concerns has affected areas of public health.

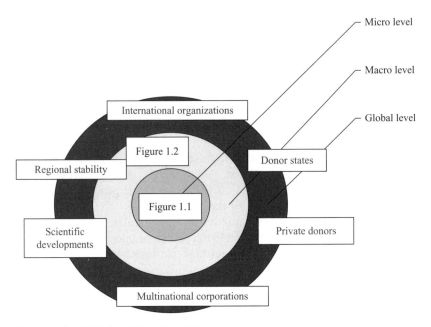

Figure 1.3   Global politics of health

It has become important, therefore, not to focus exclusively on states because a range of non-state actors play important roles in shaping access to health (see figure 1.3). One way of understanding the relationship between micro and macro factors is to approach the subject in a global context as suggested by Kelley Lee (2003). This means recognizing that we now live in a context where the actors and factors that determine our health are not shaped by strict linear relationships between individuals, doctors, states and the international realm, but interact in myriad ways depending on the context. As Kelley Lee and others have argued, the forces of globalization have led to an amalgam of actors shaping health funding, policy and provision – including international organizations, public–private partnerships, multinational corporations and civil society organizations. In this context understanding the political, social and economic forces that constitute health is important because these forces can result in individuals, states, non-state actors and international organizations reacting in very different ways to similar phenomena (see e.g. Checkel 1998).

Linking International Relations with health

At the discipline's inception, IR was primarily concerned with the study of relations between states and the prevention of war. After World War I, so-called idealists sought ways of constraining war and promoting peace between states. States have remained the primary focus of International Relations ever since, but the role that other actors – individuals, civil society groups, international organizations and corporations – play in the international 'system' (Waltz 1979) or 'society' (Bull 1977) has increasingly become part of the discussion, due to their evident impact on states and societies. As a result, the search for security and peace (or order, at least) has required a broadening of the ontology of IR. The emergence of critical security studies and constructivism, in particular, in the post-Cold War era has heralded a broadening and deepening of international relations and engagement with questions about how we understand what security is, what peace looks like and how conceptions of order, power, identity and interests are constructed and change (Walker 1997: 64–65). Today, refugees, women, children, education, environment and development figure in our picture of world politics (Finnemore and Sikkink 2001; Booth 2007). After all, according to many contemporary liberals, protecting the well-being of citizens is the key indicator of successful government. This does not mean that there are not still sceptics who question the value of opening up the 'high politics' of international relations to the 'low politics' of public health;[1] Roland Paris, for one, argues that we must not become so enamoured with expanding terms such as 'security' that we no longer know what we should be studying (Paris 2001). Nor does it mean that states are no longer pre-eminent in shaping the health of their citizens – differences in life expectancy across the Mediterranean Sea or Rio Grande are a testament to this. Instead, it means that a proper picture of world politics must take account of the impact of states on their citizens and their interaction with other actors on matters that affect their citizens' well-being.

With the broadening and deepening of IR over the last twenty years, two main ways of understanding the relationship between international politics and health have emerged. I label them 'statist' and 'globalist' perspectives, but they have much in common with securitization and critical security theories respectively. Both perspectives, which are more modes of thinking and prioritization than cogent theories, acknowledge the place of health in world politics. It should be noted that these perspectives are heuristic; they are not fixed theories with their own band of followers – or 'academic gangs', to use Colin Wight's (2004) term) – and individual writers might exhibit both statist and globalist tendencies at different times.

As its name suggests, the *statist* perspective focuses on the role of states and seeks to understand the place of health in foreign and defence policies. This approach asks how states can best respond to the threat of disease and co-operate at the international level to reduce these threats. Statist analysis typically uses the language of security. Thus, the statist perspective holds that health issues must be addressed when they directly impact on the economic, political or military security of a state. In contrast, the *globalist* perspective has more in common with critical and human security theory, and with those who maintain that health should be conceptualized as a human right, in that it seeks a reordering of how health is understood and pursued. A globalist discourse starts with individual needs and then takes into account how global actors and structures impact on the individual's health, with factors ranging from conditions of poverty and a lack of education, up to the actions of states, and the harm caused by international organizations, multinational corporations and others. The state remains a core actor in this perspective, but globalists see the state as just one among a wide number of actors, some of which have an equally significant impact on the health of individuals. The globalist perspective holds that security must be pursued first and foremost with awareness of what makes individuals insecure. Some writers who adopt a statist perspective challenge this view and argue that individuals cannot be made secure until states have the capacity to provide vaccinations and clean water and to enforce quarantine conditions during disease epidemics (Price-Smith 2009: 3–4). As such, the statist perspective tends to prioritize national security as a precursor to good health. Globalists, on the other hand, maintain that states should not be prioritized in this way as there are a number of potential systems of governance that might better protect the health of individuals. As such, states are only to be valued if they actually improve people's lives (see table 1.1).

The remainder of this chapter will set out and evaluate these perspectives in more detail, and show how they have shaped the IR contribution to public health issues.

Statist perspective

During the 1990s, heightened awareness of the threat that infectious disease outbreaks (in particular) could pose to national health, as well as economic and political stability, encouraged IR scholars to focus on the

Table 1.1   Statist and globalist perspectives

	Statist	*Globalist*
Referent	State	Individual
Actors	State; Actors that assist or reduce state's ability to respond	Individual; State; Donor states; Neighbouring states; International organizations; Private donors; Multinational corporations; Civil society organizations
Threat	Will a particular disease threaten the state?	Who is most vulnerable to disease?
Response	Strengthening institutions that will protect the state system	Any number of actor(s) or institution(s) most likely to alleviate the impact of disease on individuals
Ethos	State is best placed to manage health threats	Anyone who alleviates the threat is best placed to manage health threats

threat of infectious diseases and led many Western governments to develop responses under the rubric of national security. Acute awareness that Western states were not immune to these threats was provoked by outbreaks such as the West Nile virus near New York City in 1999, and drug-resistant infectious diseases such as tuberculosis (TB), measles and meningitis in the United States and United Kingdom, as well as the spread of SARS (severe acute respiratory syndrome) to Toronto in 2003 (Price-Smith 2002, 2009; Fidler and Gostin 2008).

For most of the twentieth century, public health in the developed world was managed by local or national groupings, be it local councils ensuring clean water or national governments providing vaccination programmes and ensuring quarantine of infected populations. Public health was a 'low politics' issue (Fidler and Gostin 2008: 9). On the rare occasion that health policy was discussed at the international level, it was in relation to (mostly) infectious disease outbreaks such as plague and cholera, or large-scale efforts such as the mass immunization programme led by the World Health Organization (WHO) to eradicate smallpox by the later 1970s. During infectious disease outbreaks, emphasis was squarely placed on the responsibility of the host state, with international efforts focused on developing mechanisms to prevent the outbreak from spreading outside borders through mixed implementation of notification and quarantine measures, as well as the regulation of air and sea traffic (Fidler 1999). Andrew Price-Smith argues that until US President Clinton's appointment of the National Science Council on Emerging and Re-Emerging Infectious Diseases in 1995, developed states were far too complacent and failed to realize that 'despite their enormous technological and economic power, it is extremely unlikely that developed countries will be able to remain an island of health in a global sea of disease' (2002: 122). In some respects, the success of the smallpox eradication programme spearheaded by WHO had only reinforced this complacency.

The emergence of HIV in the early 1980s and recognition of its potential threat to state cohesion and national economies, as well as studies that argued military forces were particularly vulnerable to HIV infection, played a major role in introducing health to IR (Elbe 2006). The apparent potential for HIV/AIDS to cause state collapse or serious disruption, with possible failure of neighbouring states with high HIV prevalence rates, was widely thought to be a realistic scenario in Southern Africa, the Pacific and some parts of South and East Asia (Shisana et al. 2003; Ramiah 2006).

In response, a host of analysts including Peter W. Singer (2002), Robert Ostergard (2002) and Stefan Elbe (2006) called for the fields of Political Science and IR to engage more with the economic, humanitarian, political and security ramifications of the AIDS epidemic. David Fidler (1999) and Andrew Price-Smith (2002) called for IR to appreciate the impact of infectious disease (from known and unknown pathogens) on state security. Using quantitative analysis of the relationship between infectious diseases and state capacity, Price-Smith claimed that 'infectious disease constitutes a verifiable threat to national security and state power' (2002: 19). Drawing from Laurie Garrett (1996) and Dennis Pirages (1997), Price-Smith invoked the term 'health security' to warn that infectious disease had the potential to cripple developing *and* developed states. Health security, he argued (Price-Smith 2002: 9, 15), referred to the threat of a country's economic and political stability being rendered unsustainable as a result of a pathogen wiping out the core population base.

In a similar vein, David Fidler's seminal 1999 book, *International Law and Infectious Diseases*, insisted that with the increased risk of drug-resistant microbes in the twenty-first century, as identified by public health officials (Institute of Medicine 1992; Heymann 1996), it will become important to 'understand the international politics of infectious disease control, or *microbialpolitik*' (1999: 19). Microbialpolitik, argued Fidler, is 'wrapped up not only in traditional concerns such as sovereignty and power but also in the implementation of scientifically sound infectious disease policies at the national and international levels' (1999: 19). It is the product of '(1) the impact infectious diseases have on international relations, and (2) the impact the structure and dynamics of international relations has on infectious diseases and their control' (ibid.).

Both Fidler and Price-Smith argued that the risk from newly emerged infectious diseases and drug-resistant infectious organisms required that governments engage with them as if they were threats to national security. In 2001, Price-Smith drew together a number of analysts to document 'the emergence of disease . . . [as] a growing threat to national security in both the developing and developed world' (2001: 3). He argued that the threat lies 'wherein the emergence and re-emergence of infectious diseases constitutes a direct threat to the lives and welfare of populations, endangering national security' (Price-Smith 2001: 4). Since then, Price-Smith has conducted a study on the fear of contagion, and argued that contemporary debates about the securitization of health issues ignore the historical context where polities in the past 'clearly perceived pathogens as profound threats to their material interests, their power, and often their survival' (2009: 207). Therefore, according to Price-Smith (2009: 207), there needs to be a reconceptualization of national security that includes non-anthropocentric threats such as naturally occurring epidemic disease. Likewise, Laurie Garrett argued in 2001 that 'a sound public health system, it seems, is vital to societal stability and, conversely, may topple in the fact of political or social stability or whim. Each affects the other: widespread political disorder or antigovernmentalism may weaken a public health system, and a crisis in the health of the citizens can bring down a government' (Garrett 2001: 5).

These ideas have permeated the politics of health and have been adopted, to some extent, by WHO. For example, WHO's 2007 *World Health Report* basically accepted the statist emphasis on linking health to security by arguing:

> Collaboration between Member States, especially between developed and developing countries, to ensure the availability of technical and other resources is a crucial factor not only in implementing the [International Health] Regulations, but also in building and strengthening public health capacity and the networks and systems that strengthen global public health security. (WHO 2007b: 13)

Encapsulating this theme, Christian Enemark maintained that 'the best candidates for securitization are those infectious disease threats that inspire particular human dread, and which therefore generate a level of societal disruption disproportionate to the mortality and morbidity they pose'

(2007: 1). While acknowledging the potential dilemma in using securitization discourse to engage the public in recognizing the risk of particular infectious diseases at the expense of a more pragmatic perspective, Enemark maintained that the 'value of securitization is that it promises to attract greater political attention and resources for protecting human health and human lives in the face of specific infectious disease threats' (2007: 20).

Overall, such an argument ultimately rests on the view that states and international organizations (e.g. United Nations Security Council [UNSC], WHO, WTO) are more likely to take health issues seriously if they are presented as national security threats similar in type to nuclear proliferation by rogue states. As I will highlight later, some globalists argue that emphasizing securitization as a solution to health crises can potentially divert attention away from the most deadly diseases and their causes by drawing attention only to those problems that have 'headline grabbing' qualities. Securitization requires shared agreement about the source of an existential threat and involves a particular logic involving the identification of threat sources and referents (Buzan et al. 1998b). This makes it well suited for addressing acute crises, but less well suited for chronic health crises (McInnes and Lee 2006; Collier and Lakoff 2008). Identifying bioweapons along with pandemic influenza, for example, as health security threats will facilitate policies to prevent these particular health crises, but it may not alleviate the underlying causes of infectious disease – which include poverty and poor health care in developing countries – and may even draw resources away from these areas. While these factors often create the conditions for pathogens to spread and to develop antibiotic resistance, they are not easily securitized (McInnes and Lee 2006). Nor are all cases of poor health that affect large numbers of the world population the result of communicable disease.

There are three other important points to note at this stage. First, by using the language of security in traditional terms, statists introduce an 'inside/outside' dynamic that may be unhelpful in relation to health. Walker (1993) argues that security has been traditionally associated with structures of friend and foe – there is an inside to protect and an outside to protect against. In this case, many statists still see states as the primary referent as well as the principal actor. The role of the state is to protect itself and its citizens from threats that come from the outside. To give a specific example, Jeremy Youde (2005) argues that neorealist, neoliberal and constructivist theories of International Relations need to engage with health issues, specifically HIV/AIDS, because health security advocates have largely failed to 'make explicit references to traditional security studies paradigms or international relations theories' (Youde 2005: 197).

AIDS can be a threat to armed forces, to the economy and to political stability on the *inside* and at the same time the existence of AIDS in the region can destabilize other states not yet affected by the illness, and thereby create regional disorder on the *outside* (Youde 2005).

While the statist perspective calls for a new security discourse where health is prioritized, it still relies on traditional understandings of what constitutes a threat and how threats should be conceptualized. Thus, they attempt to make AIDS or pandemic influenza a threat tantamount to a foreign enemy that must be vanquished or contained. This is an obvious oversimplification; nonetheless, there is a generalized perception that securitization is a useful strategy for elevating health as a policy priority in international relations (Peterson 2006). Authors such as Bower and Chalk (2003), Price-Smith (2002), Kelle (2007) and Fidler (2007b) advocate (particular) health issues in the language of traditional security concerns. Very often, their emphasis is on the state as the referent that can be rendered insecure by a health threat – usually infectious disease or bioterrorism. Those parts of the state considered most vulnerable are the military, the economy and political structures. The best way of responding to the threat, statists typically argue, is for individual states to develop health security policies, strategies and capacities.

The second key point about the statist perspective is that it focuses *overwhelmingly* on infectious disease – especially HIV/AIDS, MDR TB (multidrug-resistant tuberculosis), pandemic influenza, and bioweapon pathogens. This is interesting because, according to the Copenhagen School's theory of securitization, for issues to be defined as security issues they have to 'meet strictly defined criteria that distinguish them from the normal run of merely political. They have to be staged as existential threats to a referent object by a securitizing actor who thereby generates endorsement of emergency measures beyond rules that would otherwise bind' (Buzan et al. 1998b: 5). Infectious disease best fits this requirement because it is the health problem most likely to constitute an emergency requiring intensive short-term intervention by states. Just consider a few of the quotes that exemplify the statist perspective in their description of infectious disease in the health security context:

> AIDS not only threatens to heighten the risks of war, but also multiplies its impact. The disease will hollow out military capabilities, as well as state capacities in general, weakening both to the point of failure and collapse. (Singer 2002: 145–146)
>
> [T]he actual and potential dangers associated with microbial agents extend well beyond the relatively parsimonious *realpolitik* assumptions and paradigms, carrying direct implications for broader human, political and socioeconomic considerations. (Chalk 2006: 129)

As we can see, the speech act concentrates on a 'problem' that is uncontrolled, pervasive and a 'threat' to the very core of national security, that 'an essential trust, between government and its people, in pursuit of health for all has never been established' (Garrett 2001: 12). Authors such David Fidler and Lawrence Gostin (2008) argue that this is why collective efforts are required to prevent an inevitable river of microbes coming our way. However, this call to action could quickly become vested in self-interest and the logic becomes one of preventing 'external' problems entering the state's territory. According to this view, assistance should be provided to developing states to help 'fix' their health infrastructure because it protects states that are presently 'secure' from these pathogens in the long run. It is no coincidence that this perspective focuses on infectious disease. However, in resorting to infectious disease as the starting point for the 'call to arms' with the hope or expectation that it will lead to overall improvements in health care delivery, advocates could be destined to failure. As Peterson (2006: 46) argues, 'appealing to the national interest of advanced industrialized states like the United States to justify a massive commitment to international disease control will likely fail, because the true security implications of IDs [infectious diseases] for the United States remain limited and indirect'. The securitization premise 'relieves Westerners of any moral obligation to respond to health crises beyond their own national borders' (Peterson 2006: 46). Of course, securitization of health also fails to improve our understanding of why particular infectious diseases escalate 'out of hand' in the first place and may do little to mobilize a global effort to help those most affected (Bingham and Hinchliffe 2008).

Colin McInnes (2004: 53–55) contends that the securitization argument elevates the status of infectious disease to the point where it has created impetus for resources and international attention to be focused on the prevention of outbreaks in the developing world. The existential nature of the threat makes infectious disease a legitimate focus for world attention, and securitization is a useful strategy for making the case for extra resources. This position is certainly not without merit, but the statist case has not yet succeeded in delivering significant amounts of money or new resources to prevent the threat of disease in the first place. Rather, responses are still primarily focused on developed states protecting their own (McInnes and Lee 2006). Recently, Fidler has argued that maintaining health as a foreign policy issue is vulnerable due to two tensions. The first is complacency: to engage health at the foreign policy level requires crisis escalation – but as the selected crisis passes, public health prevention and protection will be neglected again (leaving everyone vulnerable to the next health crisis). Second, health policy improvement requires many areas to collaborate, which means that it is pushed down the list and 'subordinates health to other non-health problems and crises' such as global economic crisis and climate change (Fidler 2009: 29). The argument that infectious disease constitutes an emergency requiring extraordinary measures indicates that, overall, individual health is not actually being seen as a referent object. In line with the broad statist perspective, the securitization of health focuses on national-level threats rather than treating an individual's health as an end in itself.

The third point about the statist perspective is that there is an inherent contradiction in that, while it focuses on states as agents and referents, it also maintains that infectious disease is a transboundary phenomenon that cannot be alleviated by individual states alone. For example, Fidler (2005) calls for international law to *bind states* to take collective action against infectious disease. David Fidler discusses how states have collectively realized that the threat of infectious disease outbreaks requires increased co-operation, as demonstrated when the revised International Health Regulations were universally passed in the World Health Assembly in 2005 (see chapter 6). Fidler argues that this increased co-operation is representative of states' awareness that relying on traditional Westphalian concepts of sovereignty to protect oneself from infectious disease no longer works. States realize that they must now co-operate in a 'post-Westphalian era' because infectious disease spreads regardless of state borders (Fidler 2004c, 2005). In a similar vein, Price-Smith (2002), Youde (2005) and those concerned with the impact of AIDS (Ostergard 2002; Elbe 2006) argue that the traditional *realpolitik* of state self-help will not address the problems they identify. But at the same time, those who advocate global governance solutions do not reject the need for states to remain the key security referent (Buzan et al. 1998).

According to the statist perspective, therefore, the health of individuals requires effective state structures. Although this perspective recognizes the need for multilateral responses to some health crises, its central premise remains focused on securing the state and employing arguments thought likely to galvanize governments into action at the international level (Buzan et al. 1998: 36). The fact that infectious disease is the health threat most often referred to further demonstrates two important points in this regard. First, that what is perceived by one state as a security threat may not be perceived the same way by its neighbours (Buzan et al. 1998: 34). In the area of infectious disease this is a particularly important point to note. Countries such as those in sub-Saharan Africa and Asia cope with a number of infectious diseases. To suddenly ask these states to take a securitized view of one particular disease, e.g. influenza, is to ask them to adopt new priorities that may not fit with their own perception or the reality of their state's health needs. The second point is that there is little direct correlation between what is securitized and the health issues that actually shorten most people's lives.

Despite progress in persuading Western governments to recognize the importance of health security (Price-Smith 2002) or biosecurity (Fidler and Gostin 2008), there has been much less movement in other areas, such as acting on UN Security Council Resolution 1308, which identified HIV as a potential threat to international peace and security (Patel and Tripodi 2007: 107). Similar to Sue Peterson, my concern is that 'security provides a relatively poor rationale for addressing health threats like AIDS' (2006: 55), and also that powerful actors still only see a health crisis as worth responding to when it threatens them. Massive national expenditure on disease control can be justified only when governments can draw a link between the threat, infectious disease, and national security.

Despite these concerns, the statist approach has been relatively success-ful in maintaining that there are health issues which deserve international political attention and analytical investigation. The problem is that in order to get health issues onto the table in foreign and defence ministries, the statist perspective has adopted a securitization approach that may not be suited to this particular area. There is no real 'shaking up' of the tra-ditional understanding of security which rests on the logic of insiders and outsiders described earlier (Walker 1993). This approach might obscure or ignore the fact that the majority of AIDS victims this decade will be young females (MacNaughton 2004: 5), and that the majority of Ebola haemorrhagic fever cases have been among isolated, displaced popula-tions in the Democratic Republic of Congo (DRC) and Uganda. Essen-tially, the rhetoric and logic of statist security does not always allow investigation and awareness of how a local issue can lead to an interna-tional health crisis. To be fair, this may be because in cases such as Ebola outbreaks in DRC there are too many other complicating factors affecting disease containment and the priority thus becomes border containment. Albeit perhaps unintended this perspective can reduce health security to a matter of basic survival and, I would suggest, the prioritization of some people over others. Moreover, the securitization approach prompts a focus on protection and containment rather than tackling root causes (Buzan et al. 1998: 207), and makes it ontologically difficult to then suggest that other public health issues (which are not infectious in nature) still deserve serious international engagement. The conditions that contribute to such high levels of communicable disease in developing countries – poverty, lack of education, inequalities in the economic system, political disenfran-chisement – also have the potential to be lost from sight in the pursuit of protecting the state and in the logic of securitization. This approach carries with it the risk that the resources needed to tackle the root causes of disease and poor health will be reallocated to insulate states from the threat of infectious disease.

Globalist perspective

The globalist approach is based on two ideas. First, that the appropriate referent should be individual humans, no matter where they live. Second, that the purpose of studying health from an IR perspective is to promote health equity: that is, for everyone to enjoy similar health resources and access to health care. These ideas are somewhat grounded in critical theories of security. Critical security theory can be described as an attempt to broaden and deepen security (Booth 2007: 31). According to this perspective, the individual is the appropriate referent of security and the focus should be on threats that endanger individuals rather than the state. This means that in some situations the state itself may be seen as posing a greater threat to individuals than other threats. By recognizing that what counts as a security issue is socially constructed, critical security theorists highlight that the meaning of security and what it applies to involves the prioritization of certain voices and issues over others. Critical security seeks to redress the imbalance by giving voice to the security concerns of those who are often excluded.

Those supporting the normative goals of critical security studies in the area of health most often evoke the term 'human security' to highlight that it is humans and not states that are the most appropriate referents of security (Thomas 2000). Briefly, it must be mentioned that there is a distinction between those who see human security as a minor widening of national security agendas and those who insist that it entails nothing less than the replacing of the state with the individual as the *primary* referent of security. Globalists tend to fall squarely into the latter category. As argued by Thomas (2000), Axworthy (2001) and Booth (2007), the human security perspective seeks to prioritize the security of humans, and in this instance their health, because their humanity is the categorical imperative. The UNDP first proposed the founding principles for human security in its 1994 *Human Development Report*, arguing that:

> For too long, the concept of security has been shaped by the potential for conflict between states. For too long, security has been equated with threats to a country's borders. For too long, nations have sought arms to protect their security. For most people today, a feeling of insecurity arises more from worries about daily life than from the dread of a cataclysmic world event. (UNDP 1994: 3)

In discussing human security from a health perspective, authors such as Caroline Thomas (1989, 2003), Obijiofor Aginam (2004, 2005a), Thomas Pogge (2004, 2005) and Paul Farmer (1999, 2005) argue that we do *not* need more statist-based global health governance but to 'radically rewrite the regulations of the global health governance agenda' (Thomas 2003: 191). The problem is not with making existing local, national and global structures stronger and more responsive to health, but to actually question how these structures have produced so much health inequality and insecurity, and to make the case for dramatic reform (Orbinski 2007). Sadako Ogata and Amartya Sen led the Human Security Commission established in 2001, defining another important milestone for the human security project in proposing that it was often the *state* that posed the greatest source of threat to its own people (Ogata and Sen 2003: 2). Thus, a number of scholars applying the globalist perspective take a decisively critical view of existing health governance structures.

Despite the evident potential of this approach, there has not been much growth in this area in recent years. Its stagnation is primarily due to pragmatic considerations. A radical reworking of the global health system – including the state – is unlikely. Instead, change will be incremental, prompting analysts to concentrate on the relatively minor reforms that might make marginal improvements. As such, analysts and advocates tend to seek to advance their cause by working within predominant structures rather than trying to create new modes of governance. Thus, Ilona Kickbusch (2003, 2004) and Thomas Pogge (2004, 2005), among others, agree that there is a need to concede that progressive reform will require assistance and co-operation from existing actors and structures – *especially* the state. Therefore, the key is to think about how existing actors and structures, from states to international organizations to private donors, can be galvanized into acting on behalf of the voiceless and vulnerable, without succumbing to the logic of securitization. To do this, the globalist approach has tended to focus on human rights (see chapter 3).

For example, Obijiofor Aginam (2005a) and Paul Farmer (1999, 2005) have demonstrated through in-depth case studies on malaria, TB and AIDS that political and economic power is crucial for deciding who is treated for what, where and when, and for how much. They contend that power can only be mitigated by arguing that everyone has a basic human right to health. Farmer argues that the solution lies somewhat in a compromise between pushing the state to continue to provide basic (health) services and civil society supplying care when it is not otherwise available (2005: 244–245). The result is imperfect, but Farmer argues that health inequity – the real cause of poor health – can only be reduced by concerted action rooted in human rights. Thus, Farmer argues that 'by arguing that we must set standards high, we must also argue for redistribution of some of the world's vast wealth' (2005: 245).

For his part, Aginam (2005a: 13) has attempted to elaborate how human rights can be used for 'bold claims to universal protection of human rights and the enhancement of human dignity' and that it is 'indispensable in reconstructing the damaged public health trust in the relations of nations and peoples'. Like Farmer, Aginam uses human rights as the framework through which all health programmes and initiatives should be constructed. Both argue that the best way to make the case for treating the individual as the primary referent for health is to promote the logic of human rights rather than the logic of security. However, as I argue in chapter 3, there are significant problems associated with the right to health, including a lack of clarity about what the right entails and who is responsible for delivering it.

In sum, the globalist approach asks what makes humans insecure and how can those insecurities be addressed. In contrast to the statist view, the state is valued only to the extent that it facilitates human security. Thus, not all 'globalists' have sought to radically alter existing political structures. In fact, some have argued that the importance of having a global health governance framework is that global actors can 'step in' when the state is failing to address human insecurity. This has led to projects that examine how global governance frameworks shape some health projects in lieu of (or in spite of) the state – such as the WHO framework convention on tobacco control (Wipfli et al. 2001; Taylor et al. 2003; Yach et al. 2007), the polio eradication campaign (Aylward et al. 2003; Kirton and Kokotsis 2007), and the less successful attempts to promote gender equity (Lush and Campbell 2001; Doyal 2005), AIDS treatment (Lee and Zwi 2003; Barnett 2006) and tuberculosis prevention and treatment (Porter et al. 2002; Kim et al. 2003). As I mentioned earlier, the number and type of health actors has risen exponentially in the past few decades. However, the globalist approach seeks to understand the role of various actors in global health governance, and to gain a critical understanding of how global health governance has emerged and operates (Woodward et al. 2001). What unites the globalist perspective, and makes it distinct from the statist perspective, is the argument that health insecurity cannot be understood through the prism of the state alone.

Of course, this globalist position has not been without its critics. Stephen Walt has argued that broadening security to include all humanity rather than specific threats to states is impractical and dangerous (1991). The role of security, critics like Walt assert, is to assist the state to maintain peace, and prevent and prepare for war. Defence forces are not there to treat diarrhoeal disease, but to secure borders and forward plan for the defence of the state. Broadening security beyond traditional national security reduces its coherence and utility, and is a distraction from the real threats that make populations vulnerable. In a different vein, Fred Halliday has pointed out that the critical IR literature needs to be careful about 'making broad claims about how the international system ought to operate, with precious little indication of how practical or realistic this might be' and that in the area of issues such as foreign aid and migration (health is not referred to but we can assume it is also in danger) 'one is often hard pressed to identify anything other than claims about morality in what is being said' (1996: 326). Likewise, as mentioned earlier, Roland Paris (2001) warns of the potential for human security to be nothing more than 'hot air' unless more empirical work is done to back up the normative argument for placing humanity at the centre of security analysis. If security becomes everything, it simultaneously becomes nothing as it loses its analytical value.

There are also grounds for arguing that globalists exaggerate the extent to which the state is being replaced by other actors and underestimate the continued importance of the state in responding to health issues that concern them. There are few consistent empirical findings to demonstrate that in the area of health the state has less influence than actors such as the Gates Foundation or WHO. Indeed, the power of sovereigns to determine the well-being of their citizens leads some critical security scholars to lament the lack of progress beyond the 'business as usual' of the state system (Booth 2007: 326–327).

Where next?

These criticisms aside, the statist and globalist perspectives are both right to point to a dramatic expansion of global health governance (Buse et al. 2002; Lee 2003; Fidler and Gostin 2008). This is best illuminated in three key texts produced by different arms of the United Nations at the turn of the century, all attempting to understand how to progress the globalist perspective further, particularly the human security approach. The UN Secretary-General's High Level Panel on Threats, Challenges and Change put forward a new case for collective security in 2004, arguing that '[T]oday, more than ever before, threats are interrelated and a threat to one is a threat to all' (High Level Panel 2004: 14). The Panel argued that poor (or ill) health should be considered as a security threat because it is unlimited in whom it can threaten. In September 2000, the UN Millennium Summit brought together some 180 states to decide on development goals that all states should have met by 2015. World leaders agreed that one of the eight Millennium Development Goals (MDGs) was that health for all should be achieved by 2015 in the specific areas of controlling epidemic infectious disease, reducing child mortality, providing access to safe drinking water and adequate food to combat preventable disease, and reducing the mortality rate of women in childbirth (UN 2007). A Commission on Macroeconomics and Health for the United Nations was set up in 1999 with the intent of determining how to achieve the health-related MDGs. Its core findings, released in 2001, were that 'the massive amount of disease burden in the world's poorest nations poses a huge threat to global wealth and security' (Brundtland 2003: 419). It also found that millions of impoverished people died of preventable and treatable infectious disease because they lacked access to basic health care and sanitation, and the morality and morbidity rate could be changed if wealthier nations provide poorer countries with health care and services (Sachs 2001: 2). The MDGs were therefore seen as an attempt to prioritize the health of the world's poor.

The MDGs, the UN Secretary-General's High-Level Panel on Threats, Challenges and Change and WHO documents such as *Global Defence against the Infectious Disease Threat* (Kindhauser 2003) all represent an attempt to abandon traditional notions of sovereignty and Rob Walker's 'inside/outside' distinction discussed earlier. They seek to promote collective responsibility for health and a recognition that health threats are not characterized by state boundaries but by what threatens individuals – including poverty, environmental degradation and preventable communicable disease. The statist approach has had some success in creating global awareness of the need for wider ideas of security, while the globalist approach has had some success in promoting thinking about security from the 'bottom up' (Booth 2005: 268).

Partly as a result of the statist perspective's success in gaining world attention, those who aspire to a globalist perspective have begun to tailor their arguments in statist terms. For example, the UN reports on health security discussed above used statist arguments, referring to the threat that would be posed to developed nations if they failed to deal with health problems in the developing world. The reports used the discourse of an 'existential threat' and not just because people everywhere should not die from preventable disease, but because 'the massive amount of disease burden in the world's poorest nations poses a huge threat to global wealth and security' (Sachs 2001) in the developed world. Also because 'the security of the most affluent State can be held hostage to the ability of the poorest State to contain an emerging disease' (High Level Panel 2004: 14); and finally the 'strengthening of global capacity for routine disease surveillance and outbreak response is an essential component of preparedness for a possible attack using biological weapons . . . In some national security circles, this approach is regarded as a wise "dual use" investment that prepares for a potential security threat while also providing a clear public health benefit' (Kindhauser 2003: 17).

In essence, these positions are not dissimilar to the statist approach: in order to galvanize action, it is essential for developed states to realize that the threat of people dying from infectious disease in the poor world is a threat to them (Price-Smith 2002: 72). Even ensuring better public health for the poor has to be presented as a potential long-term contribution to the defence of developed nations against bioterrorism and pandemics. It is only by actors such as WHO and the UN Secretary-General calling on everyone in the world to feel the 'intersubjective existential threat'[2] posed by infectious disease, that globalist ideas begin to resonate on the world stage.

This dilemma is also apparent in the recent *One World, One Health* Strategic Framework presented by international organizations (including the Food and Agriculture Organisation (FAO), World Organisation for Animal Health (OIE), WHO, UN System for Influenza Coordination, UNICEF and World Bank) in October 2008. The *One World, One Health* strategy calls for the co-ordination of global efforts to prevent human influenza by controlling H5N1, increasing investment in rapid detection of the disease and 'ensur[ing] the continuity of essential services and systems' (FAO et al. 2008: 8) to mitigate the impact of a pandemic on society, systems of governance, public health and the global economy. While the strategy refers to poverty as a key contributing factor in the likelihood of animal–human disease transmission (ibid. 16–17), of the six recommended shifts to address the risk of emerging infectious diseases only one seeks to address the concerns of the poor (ibid. 18). Globalist imperatives are evident in the framework's focus on the 'global public good' and calls for engagement to shift the focus from the protection of one state to protecting individuals everywhere (FAO et al. 2008: 21). However, it is also clear that the framework's globalist aspirations depend on the commitment of states, and the state still remains a primary actor. Therefore, it is not clear to what extent calls for global initiatives through global governance frameworks can supersede national governments when it comes to delivering *direct care* for individuals.

Even if states accept the aspirations of *One World, One Health*, voluntarily or not, the sovereign state remains the last bastion of responsibility in every case. Even if opening up the realm of actors can open up greater health possibilities, and there is evidence that increased interaction might simply expand the potential for the world's rich to exploit the world's poor to satisfy their own health and economic interests, advocates are still left needing to negotiate progressive ideas within existing structures. In this context, why should we think that simply adding more actors and initiatives to the mix will improve the delivery of health care?[3] This debate demonstrates that we are a long way from consensus on the view that humans are the primary referent of security, let alone on what this might mean in practice.

Conclusion

In this chapter I have presented two main perspectives on the relationship between health and international politics. The statist perspective uses the language of security to promote health as an issue comparable to foreign and defence policy. It highlights how weak states make poor protectors of their citizens' health, whereas stable governance makes for good health. By using securitization, the statist perspective seeks to elevate health issues to the realm of 'high politics'. Therefore, the statist account often presents health issues, such as infectious diseases, as being equivalent to national security threats. As will be discussed in chapter 6, this perspective focuses on particular health concerns such as AIDS or pandemic influenza, in order to invoke traditional security understandings of what constitutes a threat. As a consequence, health concerns that do not elicit the same fear or concern as those that can easily evoke 'threat language' can be lost in the statist perspective. In contrast, the globalist perspective focuses on individual health needs and on how the state may or may not be meeting these needs. The globalist approach does not assume that the state is necessarily the most significant or legitimate actor for delivering health care to individuals. The globalist perspective tends to acknowledge a broader variety of health concerns because it is primarily interested in the issues that affect most people rather than the health issues that could affect the security of the state apparatus. The problems for this perspective are that it can lead to downplaying the importance of states and with broadness comes a lack of analytical clarity.

Regardless of these concerns, to some extent statist and globalist approaches have converged to frame how we think about the international relations of health. As will be discussed in the chapters that follow, there is an underlying tension in ensuring that health issues receive the attention of those engaged in 'high politics' without compromising the needs and rights of individuals. In practice, little progress has been made without calling on traditional statist concerns and without representing health problems as potential threats to security and stability. While this might make sensible politics in the short term, it is important to acknowledge the inherent dangers in this approach. Not least, it has the potential to skew priorities away from tackling the root causes of health problems towards a short-term approach focused only on containing particular infectious diseases.

2 GLOBAL HEALTH ACTORS

This chapter surveys the range of different actors presently engaged in the global politics of health. As discussed in the previous chapter, statist and globalist perspectives have both highlighted the dramatic expansion of actors, and the phrase 'global health governance' has been coined to explain their interaction (Cooper et al. 2007). This chapter seeks to identify these actors and to understand the way in which they function in order to better understand the global context for the issues explored in the remainder of the book.

The development of the Weberian state saw the evolution of bureaucracies dedicated to the administration of health services. All 192 member states of the United Nations and World Health Assembly have a Ministry of Health in one form or another. This implies that each state takes some responsibility for the health of its citizens, or at least attempts to administer services that will address its citizens' health. The quality of care and the depth of bureaucratic reach depend on political engagement as well as economic capacity. However, at the same time, many states rely on foreign aid to provide health care for their citizens and approximately US$6 billion a year is given in donor grants to low-income countries. Yet, as Jeffrey Sachs has argued, this is not enough. Instead, $66 billion needs to be invested in low-income countries just to address *essential* health needs, and if such an investment was made, by 2015/2020 it could generate economic benefits of $360 billion per year (Sachs 2002: 1; WHO 2002: 12–13). In addition to the role of states in managing the provision of public health care, Sachs also identifies donor states as playing a crucial role in determining what level of care is provided to individuals in the countries that are reliant on foreign aid. Furthermore, economic, societal and technological factors increasingly impact on the health of individuals through their own choices or the choices made by a state in managing its citizens' health (Yach and Bettcher 1998a; McMichael and Beaglehole 2000; Ghobarah et al. 2004; Ruger 2007). The impact of various actors on an individual's health can be thought of in terms of hubs and spokes – with the spokes (health events) impacting on the hub (individual) (see figure 1.2 in chapter 1). What is new today is the sheer number of actors and influences that an individual can be exposed to, which shape their health prospects and their access to health care.

This chapter will unfold in three parts. First, it will chart the emergence of 'global health governance' and reasons why such a term has come into existence. Second, the chapter maps the evolution of different types of health actors, focusing first on some of the most influential international organizations such as WHO and the World Bank,[1] and the increased role of non-state actors, including humanitarian and philanthropic agencies. Finally, the chapter will trace the role that remains for donor and aid-recipient[2] states in the area of global health governance. In the final section of the chapter I consider the relative influence of these actors and the relationship between them.

Global health governance

Global health governance has been defined as concerning 'the collective forms of governance, from the sub-national to the global level, which address health issues with global dimensions' (Lee and Goodman 2002: 115). As stated in the previous chapter, both statist and globalist perspectives agree on the utility of global health governance, but for different reasons. Statists see the utility of global health governance in its capacity to co-ordinate states. Globalists, meanwhile, see global health governance as a new form of politics that transcends state sovereignty and directs the focus on individuals and their vulnerabilities.

David Fidler argues that traditional appreciations of international governance focused on the 'governance of the anarchy that prevails among States' (2007a: 2). In the era of post-Westphalian governance, some non-state actors have the financial and political clout to shape international health agendas more than some governments (as will be demonstrated below). Global health governance has therefore seen the emergence of what Fidler calls 'open-source anarchy' (Fidler 2007a: 2), where the power to shape health agendas does not just reside in states alone. The emergence of global health governance has been accompanied by the arrival of non-state actors that may be more powerful than certain states in shaping health policy. What this means for the way health agendas are developed and implemented remains uncertain. This chapter starts unpacking this problem by mapping some of the key actors and the ways in which they relate to others.

International organizations

World Health Organization

The creation of the World Health Organization (WHO) was a two-year process of drafting what would become the 1946 Constitution, signed in 1948 by 61 countries (now 192) that attended the first World Health Assembly (WHA). WHO's mandate was to assist in the 'attainment by all peoples of the highest possible level of health, defined as a state of complete physical, mental and social well-being and not merely the absence of disease or infirmity' (WHA 2006: 1). While WHO was created at the end of World War II, it had been in the making for at least a hundred years. WHO was a 'direct descendent of the health organization of the League of Nations [Permanent Health Organization], and its chief aims were to promote international co-operation in the field of health and to supply expert guidance' (Harrison 2004: 181). A century earlier, the 1851 International Sanitary Conference heard a proposal from the Spanish delegation for the creation of a permanent international health body to 'resolve quarantine disputes' (Fidler 1999: 47). Similar proposals were made at the 1874 and 1884 Conferences.

The creation of regional health organizations, such as the Pan American Sanitary Bureau (PASB) in 1902,[3] provided an important foundation for the creation of the League of Nations' health organization and then WHO (Fidler 1999: 21–57). While the original emphasis back in 1851 was on infectious disease control through collective attempts to manage quarantine and surveillance, by the early twentieth century the focus had shifted 'beyond infectious disease control' (Fidler 1999: 51). The idea of bringing other public health issues to the attention of the international community – such as nutrition advice, physical education, cancer treatment and drug addiction – was based on the concept that a harmonized response to public health would be in everyone's long-term interest (Fidler 1999: 51). However, as Fidler points out, these 'lofty aspirations' did not translate into money or authority required for the organizations prior to WHO or for WHO itself to have the impact that was expected (Fidler 1999: 51–52).

By the end of World War II, health was widely seen as important for the unimpeded conduct of trade. As a result, WHO members agreed to create a number of processes and structures most unlike any other United Nations organization. For example, WHO has its own World Health Assembly comprising representatives from each member state. The WHA approves the organization's yearly programmes and its budget and sets major policy. It has an Executive Board, with a rotating membership based on technical expertise and geographical origin, which oversees all of the WHA's decisions and the work of WHO's Director-General. WHO also has six regional offices that have a fair degree of organizational autonomy in the implementation of its programmes: Africa, Eastern Mediterranean, Europe, Pan America, South East Asia and Western Pacific.

WHO's budget is divided into a biennial core fund, which covers organizational costs, annual health programmes and medical research, and an extra-budgetary fund which takes voluntary contributions from donor states and private sources to carry out specific projects. The core budget comes from member states and is determined according to the UN assessment formula that takes into account the size of each member state's economy (People's Health Movement et al. 2005: 280). Unsurprisingly, most states contribute well below the proportion that they should, according to the assessment procedure. The United States, for example, is meant to provide 25% of WHO's core funding, but pays approximately only 80% of its share to the core fund, preferring to invest the rest into WHO's extra-budgetary fund so that it can exert more control over where its contribution is spent (People's Health Movement et al. 2005: 280). The United Kingdom and other major economies do the same. As a result, Scandinavian countries are usually the highest contributors to WHO's core fund as a proportion of their gross domestic product (GDP). Of course, because extra-budgetary funds are based on voluntary funding, these programmes will almost always be geared towards specific interests of the donor rather than global health needs. In addition, because states are seeking to justify their minimal contribution to the core fund, more discussion in the Executive Board meetings tends to be spent on financial discipline and budgets than the formulation of health policy and programmes (Koivusalo and Ollila 1997: 10; *Economist* 2006: 14). This means that the WHO core budget has to provide for primary health care initiatives, training and research, as well as fund organizational requirements, while vertical programmes that have specific target outcomes are of more interest to donors under the extra-budgetary programme (Banerji 2002: 750–753). As a result, there is a close relationship between WHO's special initiatives and the interests of key donors. It has been argued that the WHO stretches itself too thin across too many projects (*Economist* 2006: 14), constraining its small funding of $1.4 billion a year (Beaglehole 2005). Others argue that, without a net growth in its budget since the 1980s, the WHO is able to achieve a remarkable amount through its core programmes (People's Health Movement et al. 2005: 280). These financial arrangements have a large impact on WHO's programme development and its internal governance. Because contributions by member states are calculated on a sliding scale, those who donate more insist that they should have more say in decision making. For example, increased voluntary donations into extra-budgetary funds by key donor states (by the early 1990s 54% of WHO's budget was extra-budgetary funds) meant that WHO programmes were heading in one direction, while the WHA, mostly comprising developing countries, had little say over the programmes that were ostensibly organized in their name (Brown et al. 2006: 68). Not surprisingly, resentment started to boil over by the mid-1990s, creating schisms between WHO headquarters and its six autonomous regional offices (Godlee 1994; *Economist* 1998: 79–80). Recently, the headquarters attempted to repair this schism and meet demands of regional offices such as PAHO (Pan-American) and WPRO (Western Pacific) by redistributing financial resources. But this has been met with concern by some analysts who argue that such devolution will only accentuate problems regarding efficiency, accountability and competency much in evidence in some of the regional offices (McCoy et al. 2006: 2180–2181), and will lead to patchier programme roll-outs (Ruger and Yach 2005).

WHO's contribution to global health policy has proceeded through four phases. During the first phase, from WHO's establishment in 1948 to the mid-1970s, the organization focused on *technical* matters. During this phase, emphasis was placed on reducing morbidity (disease) and mortality through massive vertical programmes. According to this strategy, health care efforts would be directed at eradicating single diseases such as smallpox, or would focus on one primary health initiative such as nutrition (Koivusalo and Ollila 1997: 11, 14; Bonita et al. 2007: 269). This was a period of medical marvels. For example, penicillin proved to be a 'magic bullet' for most infections, while vaccine development was at its peak (Fidler 2003a: 144). Furthermore, the eradication of smallpox by a global programme led by WHO demonstrated the potential of medical advancements and, importantly for WHO, showed that international organizations were capable of leading large and multifaceted projects with immediate impact (Burci 2007: 584).

A new Director-General, Halfan Mahler (1973–1988), made his tenure primarily about *humanitarianism* – using the offices of WHO to advocate primary health care and health equity as the key to improve the lives of millions around the world. Mahler sought to use the legitimacy that WHO had created as a leader in technical health matters to advocate for public health policies that would improve the health welfare of all humankind. In some respects, Mahler's position was a middle ground between those who wanted WHO to focus on primary health care and those who wanted it to continue focusing on technical issues, which no doubt explains his widely acknowledged success as Director-General (Godlee 1994). He appeased developing states' demand for WHO to press donor states to fund projects that focused on developing primary health care services, which was being pushed by the Non-Aligned Movement and the Soviet Union, leading to the 1978 Alma Ata Declaration on Primary Health Care and the (some argue, unrealistic) 'Health for All in the Year 2000' statement. At the same time, Mahler sought to continue the organization's technical focus with pragmatic, low-cost interventions such as 'GOBI' – Growth monitoring to fight malnutrition in children, Oral rehydration techniques to defeat diarrheal diseases, Breastfeeding to protect children and Immunizations – with UNICEF (Brown et al. 2006: 67). Mahler advocated 'international equality and rational use of resources' (Godlee 1994: 1425), raising questions about pharmaceutical practices and pricing, which led to the creation of the Essential Medicines List (see chapter 7).[4] Along with UNICEF, Mahler challenged the food industry promotion of infant formulas over breast milk, leading to the development of the International Code on Breast Milk Substitutes (Sikkink 1986).

The 1978 Alma Ata Declaration's statement on Health for All called for the 'attainment by all peoples of the world by the year 2000 of a level of health that will permit them to lead a socially and economically productive life' (Beaglehole and Bonita 2004: 187–188). However, political opposition, particularly from the United States, meant that WHO had to quickly back-pedal on this statement. Rather than seeking comprehensive primary health care, WHO promoted 'selective primary health care targets' (Beaglehole and Bonita 2004: 187–188) that were 'pragmatic, low-cost interventions' (Brown et al. 2006: 67). Comprehensive health care involved a broad definition of health, a multisector approach and community empowerment. By contrast, selective primary health care focused on the eradication of disease, power was consolidated in the hands of health professionals with an emphasis on technical solutions relating to the prevention and management of disease, and community involvement was seen as not being required for success (Beaglehole and Bonita 2004: 188).

By the time of the 1986 Ottawa Charter for Health Promotion, the economic reality of WHO's ever-decreasing budget meant that even selective primary health care was going to be difficult to achieve, let alone the comprehensive health care projects originally anticipated at the time of the 1978 Declaration (Koivusalo and Ollila 1997: 115–117; Haines et al. 2007: 911). The 1986 Charter introduced the Health Promotion programme, following the creation in 1984 of the Healthy Cities initiative by WHO's Regional Office for Europe (Koivusalo and Ollila 1997: 118). The intention was that the Health Promotion programme, like the Healthy Cities initiative, would support city-led health promotion activities that advocated nutrition, focused on women's health, and reduced tobacco and alcohol consumption, with an emphasis on the steps that individuals need to take to improve personal health (ibid. 119). This was a clear attempt by WHO to marry continued demands for a comprehensive approach to public health with the countervailling demands for a more selective approach to funding and programme development. Reviews of the 1986 Charter were mixed. Some argued that its promotion of 'partnership building' at the individual, community and structural levels produced great successes, such as the tobacco control strategy in Canada, which led to increased tobacco prices, banning of smoking in public areas and subsidized nicotine replacement therapy (Jackson et al. 2007: 81). Criticisms of the 1986 Charter were that it failed to take account of the social, economic and political factors that determine an individual's health choices, it removed the international focus on primary health care, and overlooked the fact that different cities needed different approaches, for example, health needs in Vienna are very different to Mumbai (Beaglehole and Bonita 2004: 255; Jackson et al. 2007: 82). Regardless of such concerns, the 1986 Charter meant that the objective of 'Health for All' had all but dissipated by the late 1980s (Carpenter 2000: 336).

WHO's next phase, under the leadership of Hiroshi Nakajima (1988–1996), can be best characterized as a return to technical initiatives, but largely based on the *neoliberal* model (Carpenter 2000: 343). Neoliberalism, essentially, insists that the state must take a back seat and allow the market to do its work. There should be very little regulation of the market and every attempt should be made to free private enterprise. In the area of health, this meant that the state should deregulate public health provisions. This would enable the growth of a health market, ostensibly good for the community because competition would foster advancement, and deregulation would lead to a sustainable user-pays system wherein individuals get the health they can afford. Deregulation and a private health market would free the state from large health debts and stimulate economic growth. This model was largely based on the health care system in the United States, a system that has come under criticism for being less universal and more class-based with the result that 14% of the population, some 44 million people, have no health insurance (Navarro 1999: 216, 222; Scutchfield and Last 2003: 109).

By the late 1980s WHO's budget was frozen. The World Bank stepped in to play a leading reform role in health policy, largely under the direction of the United States and the International Monetary Fund (IMF) (Navarro 1999; Carpenter 2000). Unlike WHO, the World Bank was able to attach financial incentives to its neoliberal economic reform health packages for developing states (Breman and Shelton 2007: 221). Not surprisingly, those states already experiencing high debt, afflicted by the global recession of the early 1980s and therefore reliant on World Bank funds, generally accepted the World Bank's health package and loan conditionality (see below). In turn, WHO had to quickly adapt its health packages to help secure the deliverables that the World Bank was expecting from health care programmes. Between 1987 and 1993, the World Bank increased its role in health care financing reform. In the fiscal period 1991–1994 World Bank funding for health had increased to $1.307 billion; ten years earlier it has been $103 million (Koivusalo and Ollila 1997: 26). But it should be noted that during this time recipient countries had to provide at least half of their own funds to meet each project that the World Bank agreed to fund (ibid. 27). Therefore, in step with neoliberal reforms, states introduced user fees for patients and at the same time rolled back public sector health services.

This new approach proved highly controversial. One particular dispute between European and United States donors involved the requirement in World Bank health care packages that governments introduce user fees (Lee and Goodman 2002: 100, 114). What was noticeable was the lack of WHO involvement on this issue. The WHO leadership was simply not 'in the room' on this discussion about the consequences for public health in developing countries if a user fees system was introduced (Lee and Goodman 2002: 109, 114). While UNICEF had moved on to user fees in 1987 under the Bamako Initiative, many inside WHO remained (silently) opposed to the idea of public health becoming just another commodity (Lee and Goodman 2002: 107, 109). In the meantime, the World Bank's loans for health had surpassed WHO's entire budget by 1990. In order to survive, WHO had to start working with the World Bank's health care financing reform drive and accept the neoliberal case (Brown et al. 2006: 68).

The debate continues to this day as to whether neoliberalism and WHO's capitulation to the World Bank's health care policies through the 1990s contributed to the widened gap in health care between poor and wealthier nations (e.g. Koivusalo and Ollila 1997; Navarro 1999; Breman and Shelton 2007; McMichael and Butler 2007). However, since the late 1990s, there has been a noticeable attempt by WHO to reassert its place as the key global health actor: ushering in the fourth and present phase of WHO, *institutionalism*. Institutionalism is used in the sense that WHO reclaimed its position as a leading voice in the area of health, in particular, regaining its status as the leading agency to co-ordinate and direct global health targets (Horton 2003: 324). Appointed in 1999, Director-General Gro Harlem Brundtland led the change in placing health on the table of political leaders in discussions at New York, Geneva and wherever the Group of Eight (G8)[5] meeting was being held (Horton 2003: 323–324). She achieved this primarily through promoting a relationship between 'better health and economic development' and backing 'good investments, in terms of health gain per dollar spent' (Lee 2003: 143–144).

Under the diverse leadership styles of Gro Harlem Brundtland (1998–2003), Lee Jong-Wook (2003–2006) and Margaret Chan (2006–present), WHO has launched dozens of new initiatives with other actors – e.g. private donors such as the Gates Foundation, other UN institutions such as UNICEF and UNAIDS, donor states and occasionally NGOs – to promote global health (see Horton 2003: ch. 11; Lee 2009). WHO grasped globalization to promote its role in the area of medical and technical expertise, while utilizing its relationship with other actors to promote the social and economic precursors of good health. WHO has had some success in increasing its presence on the global stage: it persuaded world leaders to include four health goals in the MDGs. WHO also negotiated its first international legal convention: the Framework Convention on Tobacco Control formally adopted by WHA in 2003 (Taylor 2002), and then in 2005 passed revisions to the International Health Regulations (see chapter 6) through the World Health Assembly. At the same time, WHO has partnered with UNICEF and the Gates Foundation in 2000 to form the Global Alliance for Vaccines and Immunization (GAVI); is lead agency for the Roll Back Malaria Campaign, which seeks to gain greater financial and political support for malaria control programmes; and worked with UN Secretary-General Kofi Annan to create the Global Fund to Fight AIDS, Tuberculosis and Malaria (Global Fund).

While Brundtlund has been commended for reasserting WHO's role in the world of global health, concerns about WHO's lack of direction and focus continue – criticism focused in particular on the lack of substance behind Brundtland's direction for WHO. Some argued WHO was left open to charges of hypocrisy: while Brundtland raised WHO's profile by targeting tobacco companies she would not criticize the pharmaceutical sector for their failure to provide access to essential medicines (Horton 2003: 332). Richard Horton argues that 'she made a great success of politicizing WHO's work to raise health higher on the global development agenda, but this politicization was a double-edged sword, and when it looked likely to incite donor disapproval, WHO's resolve collapsed' (2003: 332).

Dr Lee Jong-Wook, who replaced Brundtland in 2003, attempted to address these criticisms of WHO's lack of leadership by confronting drug companies' unfair drug pricing and introducing the '3 by 5 program' to address the HIV/AIDS drug access problem, where WHO sought to deliver access to no-cost antiretroviral treatment for 3 million individuals in developing countries by 2005. He also supported WHO's increased role in tuberculosis control (Anon. 2004a: 80). Tuberculosis had suffered from a long history of little funding and sporadic attention by the international community (Beaglehole and Bonita 2004: 276). The *Global Plan to Stop TB* was launched in January 2006 to combat the increase of multidrug-resistant TB. However, in the case of HIV/AIDS the '3 by 5' target was not reached (Ruger and Yach 2005: 1100; Gillies et al. 2006: 1405), and the *Global Plan to Stop TB* was reported in 2007 as having a funding gap of $1.56 billion (WHO 2007c). Nonetheless, Lee promised to 'finally deliver on the promises to the poor that this world has so often failed to keep' (Horton 2003: 342). Under Lee's leadership, the Commission on Social Determinants of Health (CSDH) was set up to 'marshal the evidence on what can be done to promote health equity, and to foster a global movement to achieve it' (CSDH 2008: i). The Commission, led by Sir Michael Marmot, released its final report in 2008. However, we will never know how Lee intended to realize the Commission's goals, due to his sudden death in 2006.

WHO has also sought to re-institutionalize itself as the pre-eminent authority on poverty-reduction and disease-target initiatives involving private, public and international actors (Bonita et al. 2007: 273). Present Director-General, Margaret Chan (2006–2012), has been a strong advocate for these causes. Efforts to assist states in implementing the 2005-revised International Health Regulations (IHR) have led to WHO being lauded for reasserting its global leadership in technical health matters (*Economist* 2006). However, others argue that WHO's emphasis on infectious disease prevention gives the appearance of the organization yet again avoiding its constitutional duty to create a governance framework that asserts health for all, and not just the absence of disease and infirmity (Anon. 2004b).

In response to such calls for WHO to consider its humanitarian foundations under Mahler, Chan presided over the 2008 WHO World Health Report entitled *Primary Health Care – now more than ever*, commemorating the Alma Ata Declaration and highlighting the gross health inequalities that still exist across different countries and, often, within the same country. In a speech announcing the report, Chan stated that '[T]he World Health Report sets out a way to tackle inequities and inefficiencies in health care, and its recommendations need to be heeded . . . We are, in effect, encouraging countries to go back to the basics' (WHO 2008b). Chan has been a strong advocate for the CSDH's findings, released in 2008, linking its three recommendations (improve the conditions of daily life; tackle the inequitable distribution of power, money and resources; and expand the knowledge base in the social determinants of health) to the goals of the 2008 World Health Report (CSDH 2008: 2). She has also sought to outline the obligations of donor states to address global health inequity (WHO 2008b). The question is whether WHO can generate the political and financial support required to implement the programmes necessary for primary health care delivery and to alleviate health inequity. Furthermore, there is the problem that WHO might be creating unreasonable expectations about what it can achieve.

From this brief discussion, it is clear that three problems persistently plague WHO: politics, funding and position. WHO is caught between needing to appear as a technical (as opposed to political) organization to achieve maximum funding while avoiding possible competing interests of state and non-state actors. Siddiqi (1995) may be right that WHO's greatest problems arise from politics, but politics remains unavoidable for WHO. Even if WHO reverted back to its technical phase overnight – and the present institutionalization model is perhaps the closest it has come to reverting back to this phase – states and non-state actors still appreciate WHO's work through a political lens and so do those who work within WHO. What WHO headquarters, particularly the management elite under the Director-General, choose as their mandate for the Director-General's term has political ramifications and is often rooted in political consider- ations of what will get funding and support, versus what will not. As Lee Jong-Wook said in an interview: 'WHO's role is to provide the *political* and technical leadership necessary to maintain the provision of health services, to develop and refine health infrastructure, and to implement public health standards' (emphasis added, Anon. 2004a: 79). Whichever path WHO takes there are a number of states always in opposition. As demonstrated in the early years of the 'Health for All' and Ottawa Charter debates, and more recently in the access to essential medicines debate (see chapter 7), it is rare that member states of WHO are in total agreement about the directions that need to be taken even when concerning the most technical matters of health. Furthermore, those who work within WHO are not without their own interests, and again, we see the political positions adopted by those within WHO shaping its health agenda. Thus even though the politicization of WHO may be a cause for despair for some (Siddiqi 1995), it could be argued that WHO struggles least when those within the organization appreciate the direct correlation between politics and health as a strength, rather than a weakness.

Another problem that continues to plague WHO is funding. The Bill and Melinda Gates Foundation, as well as the Global Fund, now has more financial resources at its disposal than WHO (*Economist* 2006: 14; Gillies et al. 2006: 1406). The Gates Foundation is even rumoured to be thinking about creating its 'own WHO' because, as former WHO official and head of the Gates Institute for Health Metrics and Evaluation, Christopher Murray, argues: 'a new path was needed because the United Nations agency [WHO] came under pressure from member countries. His [Gates] institute would be independent of that' (McNeil 2008). Brundtland's use of public–private partnerships (PPPs) to fund the expansion of WHO's work made it financially dependent on private organizations and bilateral agreements with states. This is a cause for continued concern. WHO's institutional independence is constrained in such relationships. In particular, WHO's engagement of pharmaceutical companies for the delivery of health programmes has been criticized because WHO is meant to function independently of corporate interests and to provide health programmes that are independently sustainable in the long term (Buse and Walt 2000a: 555, 557; 2000b: 705; Cawthorne et al. 2007: 974–975).

Finally, WHO suffers from problems of position. WHO's role in regulating health care and providing health care programmes has come under challenge from competing organizations – both within the UN system and without. The World Bank's assertion in the area of health care policy in the 1990s presented the WHO as either inert or weak; and the rise of the Gates Foundation could herald a repeat of such images (*Economist* 2008). However, WHO's role in health is 'grounded in the UN Charter' (Taylor 2004: 504). WHO is the sole authority with the 'cardinal responsibility to implement the aims of the Charter with respect to health' (ibid.). But this unique status also constrains the WHO. Some argue that the WHO needs to reconnect with its 'core duties' such as publishing national health data (*Economist* 2008). However, Taylor (2004: 505) challenges arguments that WHO should return to its traditional technical role, arguing that the organization instead needs to embrace its role as a leader in international public health co-operation on a multitude of issues.

World Bank

As we noted earlier, it has been argued that the World Bank set back health care in low- and middle-income countries more in one decade than anything that the states themselves could have done since colonialism (Koivusalo and Ollila 1997: 31–3; People's Health Movement et al. 2005: 302). Structural adjustment programmes (SAPs) that linked the deregulation and privatization of health care to development loans had a dramatic and negative effect on many developing states. In many low-income countries, health costs remain the primary source of debt for families (People's Health Movement et al. 2005: 63–64). Moreover, it is commonly argued that the rise in the burden of disease among the poor and vulnerable in countries relying on SAPs can be directly linked to the World Bank's policies because they encouraged governments to reduce health spending (Lee and Goodman 2002: 101; Breman and Shelton 2007: 230–231).

Before looking at these claims in more detail, we must understand what the World Bank is and why it was able to influence health policy to such a degree during the 1980s and 1990s (Ruger 2005). The World Bank loaned approximately $24.7 billion for 298 new operations in 2008, Africa received 23% of the total; Latin America and the Caribbean 19%; East Asia and Pacific 18%; South Asia 17%; Europe and Central Asia 17%; and Middle East and North Africa 6% (World Bank 2009). Its aim is to reduce poverty by facilitating economic growth. The Bank's decision-making structure is based on financial contributions. Basically it is a one dollar, one vote system. As a result, the United States holds 17% of the vote and by tradition appoints the Bank's president. At the other end of the scale, 47 sub-Saharan African countries have two directors on the board (out of 24) and 7% of the vote (People's Health Movement et al. 2005: 300).

The World Bank lends money and uses the collateral of existing loans to raise more loan money through the sale of bonds to private investors. As a result, the World Bank has often made large sums of money from lending by applying interest to a portion of its loans and using loan repayments as collateral for selling bonds (Koivusalo and Ollila 1997: 26). The World Bank lending portfolio shifted from infrastructure and industrial investments in the 1950s and 1960s, to agriculture and social sector investments in the 1970s, to policy-based lending in the 1980s – focusing on specific sectoral adjustment programmes, e.g. public health sector reform (Koivusalo and Ollila 1997: 29). One key reason for the introduction of SAPs was to assist governments still paying off their loans from the 1960s and 1970s by reducing overall spending on government services. The oil shocks in the 1970s and 1980s contributed to massive deficits for governments that needed to borrow heavily (on top of existing debt) to cover domestic expenses; the global economic recession left many developing countries unable to even service their debt interest repayments. The debt crisis particularly affected developing countries that had already borrowed heavily from the World Bank and, due to a combination of corruption, poor project design, a sharp rise in interest rates and low rates of economic growth, these countries were getting into deeper debt.

At the same time, WHO had been promoting the Alma Ata Declaration with its 'health for all' ambition (see above). This had been an attractive proposition for newly independent states and those starting to improve their overall economic position. However, primary health care was not cheap and 'the necessary additional resources proved not to be forthcoming, and widespread reallocation from urban hospitals to rural health facilities did not happen on any appreciable scale' (Lee and Goodman 2002: 99). In 1985, de Ferranti estimated that primary health care implementation would cost worldwide $50 billion a year (quoted in Lee and Goodman 2002: 99). This was at a time when economies, particularly developing economies, were facing severe recession due to the wider financial market crisis and ever-increasing interest rates on their national debts. As a result, developing countries simply had no additional money to spend on primary health care projects.

As WHO's Alma Ata initiative died and WHO's budget froze, the World Bank – without a clear mandate for health – came to regard itself as 'the major funding agency for population and health issues' by the 1980s (Koivusalo and Ollila 1997: 25). World Bank funding for health in the 1980s was mainly policy-based lending: loans directly linked to structural and sectoral adjustment programmes (SAPs). In the 1990s, further requirements were added: governments needed to demonstrate good governance and gender sensitivity in their programmes (Koivusalo and Ollila 1997: 29). Money directed towards health programmes required cost-effectiveness analysis, which some public health officials argued meant that communities would not be receiving the health care they needed but, rather, the type of care that cured the greatest number for the least cost (Koivusalo and Ollila 1997: 40–41). The problem with this was that recipient states no longer had ownership of the health care system that they had created; the objective was now to minimize costs rather than improve health care according to each state's distinct needs (Lee and Goodman 2002: 116). Health care rationing exacerbated social divisions when one group received better health care than others, and the privatization of the public health sector resulted in multi-class systems of health care (Koivusalo and Ollila 1997: 33). As we noted earlier, the World Bank emphasized economic and public policy restructuring according to neo-liberal principles (Brown et al. 2006: 67–68). Trade was liberalized (which meant that protections and tariffs were removed), investment and capital controls were removed, public expenditure was cut, and the World Bank loans were made conditional on the deregulation and privatization of state-owned industries. Most of the developing world had little choice but to comply with SAPs to prevent inflation and further indebtedness (Koivusalo and Ollila 1997: 28–31).

All this caused two key problems. First, indebtedness increased significantly. In fact, the global rich became richer and the global poor more indebted – strengthening the influence of discretionary funds for health (Cornia 2001: 835; Thomas and Weber 2004: 188). Second, emphasis on private health care rather than expenditure in the public sector meant that primary health care became less affordable for those most in need of it. Carpenter (2000: 345) argues that even the World Bank had to 'grudgingly acknowledge' that investment in health and education by the state for those least able to afford it provided a vital 'safety net'. However, the adjustment of World Bank programmes to accommodate this 'safety net' in the 1990s was too late as many governments were too indebted to fund them. Today in India, an average family will lose around 80% of its income to pay for health care, compared to the 25% that a family in a developed country will pay (the United States is unique among developed countries with the cost being 56%) (Kickbusch 2004: 208). By the turn of the twentieth century, Africa was spending twice as much on debt repayments as on health care, yet endured 50% of the global burden of disease and spent less than 2% of the global health resources (WHO 2007a: 19). The introduction of user fees, a key component of SAPs, led to a sharp drop in health consultations in Kenya, Papua New Guinea, Tanzania and Niger, among others, raising fears of a 'knock-on public health risk' in the areas of TB, STDs and maternal health care (Lee 2003: 143).

In 1993, the World Bank released its 1993 World Development Report (WDR), *Investing in Health*. The report proved controversial for two reasons. First, the World Bank was asserting more influence over global health policy than WHO. Critics argued that WHO, as the leading institution for global health, should be the lead institution on health policy rather than simply implementing World Bank policy – which was the widely held perception of WHO at the time (Koivusalo and Ollila 1997: 45; McMichael and Beaglehole 2000: 496). However, WHO was a co-sponsor of the 1993 report (Kumaranayake and Walker 2002: 144), indicating that perhaps the displeasure directed at WHO had more to do with concern that WHO had shifted from its 'traditional attitude' of arguing the merits for a publicly financed primary health care system towards a neoliberal stance (Carpenter 2000; Lee and Goodman 2002: 109). Second, the report introduced a cost-effectiveness analysis (CEA) to health, which emphasized the delivery of vertical health programmes based on whether the programme would be able to reduce a disease burden for minimal cost.[6] This model became an influential instrument of global health policy in developing countries over the following decade.

Investing in Health argued that if states must be involved in public health expenditure it should be done according to a 'burden of disease' framework. Public health like every other public programme, the report argued, needed to prioritize core areas of health to produce the best outcomes or a 'good buy' (Kumaranayake and Walker 2002: 145; see also n.6). Poor health always poses a cost burden to the community, but some diseases create a higher cost burden than others. To measure this, the potential years of life lost (PYLL), quality-adjusted life years (QALYs) and disability-adjusted life years (DALYs) were introduced to provide 'subjective parameters in order to value the outcome' of where public health expenditure could create the best economic outcome for a community (Musgrove 2000: 110). DALYs have proved to be most influential in World Bank policy, while the WHO takes DALYs into account when providing its yearly 'global burden of disease' studies. DALYs work on the principle that the need for a health intervention or allocation of resources to a health sector should be determined by measuring the 'standard expected years of life lost from different illnesses and conditions calculated according to different age groups, sexes and geographical regions' (Murray 1994: 431).

Although the DALY is just one of the guides that WHO uses when formulating policy, it has continued to be an influential method used by the World Bank for determining whether to fund health projects. (Musgrove 2000: 113). What is most concerning about the DALY is that it has the potential to distort health policy if it becomes seen as the 'only method in town' for determining the direction of health care funding (Lee and Goodman 2002). DALY gives, for example, less value to early childhood and older ages based on the premise that people in their early adult and middle years are more economically beneficial to the community. Nor does DALY take into account the differences in health conditions between developed and developing countries. For example, Gwatkin (1997: 141) argues that while non-communicable diseases are responsible for 56% of all deaths worldwide, communicable disease remains the largest cause of death in the developing world at 56% compared to 8% in the developed world. WHO's mandate advocates that the attainment of health is about *more than the absence of infirmity and/or disease*, yet the DALY focuses only on the absence of disease and measures intervention in terms of cost effectiveness. The focus is placed squarely on morbidity and mortality rates, and their effect on the economy. As a result, DALY skews priorities towards men within the middle age bracket, while excluding children, the elderly and women (Koivusalo and Ollila 1997: 34). The consequence, it is argued, is that the World Bank's health funding became a 'minimal package' that focused on cost effectiveness, averting only one-third of the estimated burden of disease in low-income countries and under a fifth in middle-income countries (People's Health Movement et al. 2005: 75).

In 1999, the World Bank introduced Poverty Reduction Strategy Papers (PRSPs) in an effort to correct some of the problems associated with the SAPs (Wamala et al. 2007: 234). The World Bank argued that heavily indebted poor countries (HIPCs) needed to reclaim ownership of their economic reforms, and that aid programmes were most effective when governments were able to structure them and have targets easily identified by donors. In addition, the PRSPs are a medium- to long-term loan process, which allowed for long-term forward planning. In practice, ownership in the PRSP process is still open to doubt by virtue of the interest that the World Bank and IMF have in the HIPCs (Wamala et al. 2007: 238). The continued emphasis on privatized health care has led to many arguing that the PRSPs are effectively SAPs with a different name and new conditionalities (Schrecker et al. 2007: 190). Again, however, the arrival of Gro Brundtland – who sought to promote health in the international development agenda and needed private investment and voluntary contributions to fund WHO's expanding programme – gave strong support to the PRSP process despite concerns within WHO itself (People's Health Movement et al. 2005: 274).

An outcome of the SAPs and PRSPs is that poor states are even more reliant on external funding for health than they were before the international financial reforms of the 1980s (Wamala et al. 2007: 234). An example of the impact that World Bank policies have had on health spending is the case of Tanzania. The Tanzanian government had been trying to reduce its debt for over a decade. Between 1986 and 1998, the period in which Tanzania implemented a number of World Bank sponsored programmes to reform its economy, its 'total external debt stock grew by about 62.2%, with the aggregate ratio of debt service to exports estimated at 27.4% at the end of 1998' (Nanda 2006: 194). Approximately 30% of government revenue went on servicing Tanzania's debt between 1998 and 2001, which resulted in reduced government expenditure on health and other public services (ibid.). The 2003 Brundtland Commission on Macroeconomics and Health, chaired by Sachs, found that states should spend *at least* 12% of their GNP on essential health care. The World Bank PRSP originally allowed Tanzania to increase spending from 7.5% to 8.7% of GNP on health care, but each year since the increase has declined. It appears that one impediment to increased health expenditure is that governments need to have enough tax revenue to continue this investment. This has been a problem for Tanzania because another loan conditionality of the World Bank was to liberalize trade – which has meant a revenue loss for the government of Tanzania because, as in most other developing countries, income tax revenue is too low to supplement the loss from taxes collected through tariffs on imported goods (Nanda 2006: 195). Priya

Nanda argues that one direct result of implementing the World Bank's policies has been that Tanzania's overall life expectancy fell from 50.1 years in 1992 to 43.1 years in 2002 (Nanda 2006: 194).

In summary, the World Bank is an important actor that wields immense influence over what issues are placed on the 'global health governance' agenda and this will continue into the future (Kumaranayake and Walker 2002: 153–155). To date, however, its proclivity for neoliberalism has tended to do more harm than good for enhancing public health capacity to address poor health care delivery within states reliant on World Bank lending. Even when the World Bank adjusts its investment programmes to allow governments to invest in sectors that care for those less fortunate, the core business of the World Bank – trade liberalization and high interest debt repayments – makes it very hard for governments to accommodate even a nominal health care investment. This is an area of 'global health governance' that demonstrates the impact an external actor can have on the health of individuals. Securing states from indebtedness has come at the cost of diminished public health care for their citizens. The dramatic expansion of health actors at the international level does not always herald well for individuals who cannot rely on their state for health security.

Non-state actors

There has been a shift in the politics of health from a series of vertical care delivery processes to a horizontal process, where a variety of actors work in alliances and partnerships and no longer simply rely on the 'public' sector to deliver programmes (Walt and Buse 2006: 649). However, there are questions about the accuracy of the 'public'/'private' label. Should non-governmental organizations (NGOs) and transnational companies such as Pfizer both be placed in the 'private' sphere? Walt and Buse maintain that NGOs can fall under the public–private partnership (PPP) category because of their diversity and non-state identity. Therefore, associations such as local NGOs, large multinational NGOs like Oxfam and Médecins Sans Frontières (MSF), and private foundations such as the Rockefeller Foundation, the Ford Foundation and the Gates Foundation, all count as private partners. However, Buse and Walt acknowledge that these private bodies are quite different from actors in the corporate sector – such as pharmaceutical companies – who are also listed as private partners that have increasingly entered into public partnerships with international organizations such as UNICEF and WHO (2000a: 552).

Therefore, it is important to examine not only the role that non-state actors are playing in global health governance, but also how they understand their own role within this framework. In this section I examine a number of non-state actors according to the terms that they use to define their work in health, focusing on NGOs and philanthropic organizations. The NGOs, or humanitarian agencies, that engage in public health advocacy and health care delivery will be examined first. These agencies may operate at both the national and international level, and are defined as non-government because they are constituted separately from the government of the country in which they are founded (Sphere Project 2004). I will then proceed to evaluate the emergence of powerful philanthropic agencies such as the Bill and Melinda Gates Foundation. The overall purpose here is to identify how these various agencies co-operate within various global health partnerships (Buse and Walt 2000a, 2000b), while at the same time pursuing their independent health care agendas. The role of business in the global politics of health is more closely examined in Chapter 7.

Humanitarian agencies

Articles 18(h) and 71 of the Constitution of the WHO state that the organization can 'cooperate with national NGOs *only* with the consent of the government concerned' (WHA 2006). This was not a particularly auspicious start for national NGOs as it enabled some authoritarian governments to deny NGOs with strong grassroots support the opportunity to build their profile by partnering with WHO (Litsios 2004: 61). Conversely, it is ironic to note that today WHO is often having to 'catch up' with the health care delivery and advocacy work being done by international humanitarian agencies such as MSF and Oxfam (McCoy et al. 2006: 2181–2182; Ruger and Yach 2006: 1100). Meanwhile, the level of partnerships between international NGOs and private foundations such as Rockefeller (which began almost as soon as WHO was created) has expanded exponentially. Opponents (including some within WHO) criticized the organization at the time for not adequately engaging with NGOs in the co-ordination of health care programmes in developing countries during the 1960s and 1970s (Litsios 2004). In response, Director-General Mahler invited NGOs to the Alma Ata Conference for the first time as delegates rather than observers, and NGOs were written into the Declaration as having a primary role in the programmes being developed by WHO and states. Since then NGOs have developed a compelling 'third' voice in global health governance. They have, among other things, advocated practical health initiatives and human rights in the areas of HIV/AIDS, reproductive and sexual health, children's health, affordable pharmaceuticals and primary health care (see chapters 3 and 7). They have often been the lone voice arguing for progressive change in these areas, when states have failed and WHO was unable to push these agendas forward. As shown in chapters 4 and 5, humanitarian NGOs such as MSF, Oxfam, International Rescue Committee (IRC), Save the Children and Merlin have also often been the key health actors in humanitarian emergencies and conflict zones.

A recent example of the important advocacy role played by an NGO was MSF's very public condemnation of the US and European governments' refusal to allow generic production of medicines for HIV and TB, which led to the Doha round of talks in 2001 (see chapter 7). Likewise, the epidemiological data gathered by the IRC in the Democratic Republic of Congo (DRC) has been vital for raising awareness in the international community that 'the vast majority of deaths [during the war] were caused by the destruction of the country's health infrastructure and food supplies' (Turner 2007: 3).

It has been argued that NGOs are able to achieve better advocacy for specific health matters because their mandate comes from proactive engagement with the issue, direct involvement with those most affected, and an independence from state or company interests (Warkentin 2002: 22). However, remaining independent is not without its difficulties, particularly for local organizations in the developing world that are reliant on external funds or in non-democratic countries where NGOs encounter many obstacles to their right to organize and freedom of speech. Being a large international humanitarian NGO allows a certain amount of freedom from the influence or pressure of any one state. For example, organizations such as MSF make a point of insisting that donors or political actors will not influence its mandate of 'testimony' about aggression against civilians. To ensure its independence, MSF insists on taking no more than 40% of its income from governments (Clapham 2006: 311). In contrast, the International Committee of the Red Cross (ICRC) is more readily accepted in crisis zones and enjoys good relations with most governments because of its longstanding neutrality in the delivery of health care programmes (Forsythe 2005).

This does not mean that international NGOs such as MSF, ICRC, Oxfam and World Vision are immune from critique. In particular, there is the problem of aid dependency whereby aid agencies obviate the need for states to manage projects and assume responsibility themselves (Buchanan and Decamp 2006; Dijkzeul and Lynch 2006a). A good example can be found in various vaccination programmes. For example, the Global Polio Eradication Initiative (GPEI) is an issue-based (as opposed to product-based, see Buse and Walt 2000a, 2000b) initiative involving WHO, UNICEF, US Centers for Disease Control and Prevention (CDC) and Rotary International, which aims to eradicate polio (Aylward et al. 2003:

41–42). The incidence and location of polio quickly demonstrates that it is a disease caused by poverty (Farmer 2005: 77). Polio has been eradicated in most developed countries since the 1980s; however, in the developing world it continues to rob lives and cause disability. There are only four countries that continue to report poliomyelitis infections: Afghanistan, India, Nigeria and Pakistan (Nordstrom 2006: 178). Vaccination against polio is seen as an effort to save lives by providing a service 'in countries where the government's health infrastructure fails to reach a large percentage of the population' (Waisbord 2005: 282). However, critics argue that GPEI creates a heavy reliance on non-state actors such as MSF and World Vision to conduct one-off training programmes for locals in vaccine delivery, rather than building local state capacity to improve essential primary health care (*Economist* 1998: 79; Waisbord 2005: 282–283). Advocates argue in response that part of the GPEI success has been the training of local health workers and volunteers to deliver the vaccine. Polio-endemic countries have contributed at least $1.8 billion in volunteer time between 1988 and 2005 (Aylward et al. 2003: 40). The concern remains that humanitarian actors are participating in projects that focus on dealing with one disease at a time, rather than advocating funding the development of primary health care systems. This is good for fundraising but it is not complementary to developing primary health care services across urban and rural areas, nor is it clear, in the case of the polio initiative, that eradication of a disease will resolve the root cause – extreme poverty that facilitates the spread of the disease in the first place (Farmer 2005: 89).

   In summary, while the proliferation of NGOs in the health field provides new opportunities, there are also significant challenges. Not least, there is the potential for NGOs to create aid dependence and distort local health policies to reflect the interests of external actors. This deference to external interests can work in two ways. First, if private donors give more to an NGO after positive publicity for its work on vertical programmes, then vertical programme delivery may become a core part of the NGO's work at the expense of investment in primary health care delivery. Second, if the NGO is overtly reliant on a particular donor government for its funding or a pharmaceutical company for vaccination and drug supplies, the NGO may be seen as creating aid dependence and distort local health policies to reflect the interests of external actors (Riddell 2007).

Philanthropic actors

Philanthropic actors in the area of health are not new: the Atlantic Foundation and the Rockefeller Foundation have influenced health care delivery and health care technology since the beginning of the twentieth century

(Farley 2004; Allen 2007). However, the investment provided by philanthropic actors to address primary health care problems has dramatically increased in the past few years (Reimann 2006). It is best indicated by comparing the 1998–99 expenditure of the Gates Foundation with WHO's budget. In the first half of 1999, Gates committed $100 million to the Bill and Melinda Gates Children's Vaccine Program; $50 million on a Malaria Vaccine Initiative; $25 million on an International AIDS Vaccine Initiative and $1 million on the International Trachoma Initiative (Buse and Walt 2000b: 705). Meanwhile, WHO's total budget for 1998–99 for its entire Control of Tropical Diseases programme was $29 million. The annual budget of WHO for the same year was less than $1 billion, while the Gates Foundation assets at that time were valued at $18 billion (Buse and Walt 2000b: 705). Clearly, philanthropic foundations such as the Gates Foundation will have a tremendous impact on health care delivery and health care projects.

Philanthropic actors are able to fund research projects and promote commercial sector linkages in such projects. However, the involvement of pharmaceutical companies in drug-based initiatives raises some concerns. Ostensibly, such initiatives aim to improve the condition of those with a particular health problem or to aid the delivery of health care. However, some critics question the increased role of private pharmaceutical companies in philanthropic projects. For example, the Malarone Donation Program (1996) involved Glaxo Wellcome, the British, American, Kenyan and Ugandan governments, as well as WHO, World Bank and the Wellcome Trust (Buse and Walt 2000b: 701). The project involved the donation of an inexpensive drug to treat malaria. On closer inspection, it was found that the drug's effectiveness was doubtful at best. Furthermore, the drug would be too expensive for governments to continue to use as a first-line therapy after the PPP ended and there was no proof that the drug was even necessary for first-line therapy (Buse and Walt 2002: 45).

Another example is the Global Fund for AIDS, Tuberculosis and Malaria, which is jointly managed by a UN and USAID chairperson, financed by the G8, and has philanthropic donors on its board, including the Gates Foundation and a number of pharmaceutical companies. The Global Fund aims to ensure that every project will be co-ordinated by the state seeking the funding, helping to address the problems of sustainability and capacity-building identified earlier. The purpose of the Global Fund is to establish a 'country-driven' (McCarthy 2007: 308) approach, which provides funds on a competitive basis to 'attract, manage and disburse additional resources to countries to control these three diseases' (Walt and Buse 2006: 655), and withdraw funding if the country receives poor performance reviews.

The Global Fund is innovative in that (if it ever achieves the full funding that has been pledged) it will amount to the largest global health programme which seeks to empower aid-recipient states and avoid aid dependency. However, it still shares several features in common with earlier PPPs – in particular, the targeting of specific diseases as opposed to establishing holistic health care programmes. Emphasis on targeting malaria, HIV and TB could distort health priorities so that a state may develop a comprehensive TB reduction strategy while other major issues (e.g. clean water) remain unaddressed (McCarthy 2007; SUS). As mentioned above, WHO has also come under criticism for its increased support for specific disease programme initiatives. Since 2008, the Global Fund has sought to address this criticism by introducing a new programme focused on strengthening health systems. Meanwhile, government health workers have raised concerns that they spend more time writing project proposals for the Global Fund than providing care to the sick (Walt and Buse 2006: 654–655).

It is difficult to know how effective these arrangements are because there are as yet few focused case comparisons on the successes and failures of PPPs. What can be surmised is that philanthropic actors, such as the Gates Foundation, have been crucial for placing health back on the list of G8 and global governance priorities. Furthermore, the amount of funding and private–public connections available as a result of these funding windfalls creates the opportunity for important scientific discoveries and delivery of care in harsh settings. However, philanthropic foundations, like NGOs, states and international organizations, seem to eschew independent performance evaluations. Unlike these other actors though, the financial independence of philanthropic foundations makes it easier for them to avoid evaluations of project performance against the project's aims and objectives. Yet in the last decade, these foundations have emerged as key players in setting health treatment targets alongside WHO, UNICEF, donor and aid-recipient countries. As such, it is important that their performance and contribution to the improvement of public health be open to independent scrutiny.

Although non-state actors play an increasingly important role, it is clear that the central actor that they all rely on for 'rolling out' their programmes is the state. The precise role of individual states may vary, but states of all stripes play a vitally important role. Donor states exert enormous influence over the priorities of international organizations and even some NGOs' budgets, and aid-recipient states play a major role in determining the effectiveness of aid projects. Although donor states tend to be more influential, when they work together aid-recipient states can wield significant influence over health issues and priorities. This final section of the chapter will assess the role of donor and aid-recipient states in shaping the global health agenda. In particular, it asks whether the development of international organizations, NGOs and private actors has strengthened or undermined the role of the state in the provision of health care.

States

Donor states

Global health governance has developed from an international system based on states co-operating with states, into a global society where international organizations co-operate with each other, NGOs, philanthropic foundations, multinational corporations and states in the area of health care policy and delivery. Those who describe this evolution from international to global health argue that the state is no longer the sole actor, and that different types of actors interconnect through dense and complex networks (Kickbusch 2003: 192–203). However, the emergence of these various actors should not let us forget the fact that states remain the most influential actor. States determine what they will financially and administratively commit themselves to, set health priorities and policies, and influence the extent to which their citizens' health will be affected by outside actors. As such, the state remains a powerful reality that must be acknowledged by both those who promote and those who examine global health governance.

In some respects, donor states are the most important actors covered in this chapter for the following reasons: they determine WHO's yearly programmes; the primary decisions made in the World Bank and IMF are determined by those who donate the most; the overwhelming majority of private donations to NGOs come from those who live in donor states, and for some NGOs their operational budget is supported by donor states; donor states are the headquarters for most philanthropic, medical research and pharmaceutical corporations; and a large number of grassroots NGOs based in aid-recipient states rely on contributions from donor state governments and those who live in donor states for funding (Riddell 2007).

As we noted earlier, WHO relies on voluntary funding for selective health care programmes, which is outside the annual budget, and the majority of voluntary funding comes from developed states such as the United States, Canada, the United Kingdom, Japan, Australia and Western Europe. As a result, these key donor states have the capacity to determine the health care projects that WHO will develop and promote.

Their interests therefore play a disproportionate role in shaping global health priorities.

For instance, the 'Child Survival Revolution', a joint programme by WHO/UNICEF, was funded by USAID (US federal foreign aid agency) and launched in 1982. This programme prioritized seven child health interventions: growth monitoring, oral rehydration therapy (ORT), breast-feeding, immunization, family planning, food supplements and female education; and it became known as the GOBI-FFF programme. More than twenty years later, 11 million children – 30,000 a day – still die from preventable causes (People's Health Movement et al. 2005: 69). This project had specific treatment targets, but did little to deal with the primary causes of diarrhoea among children – acute malnutrition, lack of access to clean water and absence of primary health care (People's Health Movement et al. 2005: 69). Nevertheless these initiatives remain popular because they offer immediate deliverables – number of people vaccinated, number of women breast feeding, etc. – whereas dealing with the underlying social and economic structural influences that contribute to child mortality is more expensive and a lot harder to change (Collier and Lakoff 2008: 17).

Likewise, the Global Alliance for Vaccines and Immunization (GAVI) was set up in 1999 with the goal of recovering the drop in immunization rates over the previous ten years by promoting the use of new-generation vaccines (Beaglehole and Bonita 2004: 271; Walt and Buse 2006: 665). GAVI's funding came from the Gates Foundation and donor states such as the Netherlands, Norway and United States, the initiative was assisted by UNICEF and WHO, and recipient states Mali and Bhutan were repre-sented on the Fund's executive committee. Under GAVI, recipient coun-tries were to apply for funding to support the delivery of vaccines. However, an early review showed that in sub-Saharan Africa there were 'several serious problems ranging from weakness in the cold chain necessary for effective immunization services to lack of planning for long-term financial sustainability if the GAVI funding stops after 5 years' (Beaglehole and Bonita 2004: 271). Countries asking for funds did not have the primary health care capacity to deliver the outcomes they promised. In contrast to previous vertically funded projects, GAVI attempted to reorient the rela-tionship between donor and recipient states, by empowering the latter with the assistance of international organizations and private funds. States set their own targets (not unlike the Global Fund) as a way of promoting local ownership, sustainability and capacity-building (Walt and Buse 2006: 665). However, the programme was still developed as a vertical frame-work, with funding coming from 'above' for the implementation of a single specific health outcome – increased vaccinations. Furthermore, the terms, the proposals, the judging and the aid provision under GAVI were all based on criteria established by donor states (see more on GAVI in chapter 7) (Richards 2001: 1322).

We therefore cannot ignore the political and commercial criteria that may influence how a donor state devises its aid to health care programmes. In general, we know that more aid goes to middle-income countries than to the poorest; less aid is received in large poor countries than in small poor countries, and very rarely is aid provided according to a poverty criterion (Riddell 2007: 104). If we consider the impact that this has from a health perspective, we can see that the way that donor states understand health care programmes is influenced by *distributional factors* – donor states and private corporations give according to the number of patients who would benefit from a specific treatment (Pogge 2004: 135). There is very little understanding of how these same actors and other social, economic and political factors may be *related* to the medical conditions that individuals confront in the developing world. Global economic institutions, Pogge (2004) argues, contribute to the conditions that create severe poverty and thus immunization programmes such as GAVI play an important distributional role, but donor states and other powerful actors have never grappled with *relational* concepts of distributive justice. In other words, they have yet to consider the redistribution of material goods to offset the contribution of neoliberal economies to creating absolute poverty and thus poor health.

Therefore, although they may make specific advances, health programmes that are funded by developed states and private donors tend to perpetuate the conditions that led to these specific diseases taking root in developing countries in the first place. Poverty creates the conditions for many diseases, which in turn perpetuate further poverty. Disease may affect an individual's means of income generation, which results in less taxable income for the state and disables many states from taking appropriate action to alleviate poverty. Vertical programmes that focus on vaccinations or new drugs may reduce the immediate harm but they will not remove the long-term health inequity that perpetuates these preventable illnesses.

Establishing the health care infrastructure to make these interventions worthwhile in the long run requires significant investment and support from donor states – something that the World Bank-inspired market liberalization model has assisted in steadily eroding (McPake 2002: 138–139; Blouin 2007: 94–96). Pogge (2004: 139–140) does not ignore the fact that aid-recipient states play a role in their citizens' abject poverty through corruption and undemocratic practices (see below) but he also argues that donor states perpetuate poverty and that their role in doing so is often overlooked because of the distribution of foreign aid programmes. Howson et al. (1998: 586) argue that donor states provide aid because they have a 'stake' in the health of people everywhere and this stake 'serve[s] to protect citizens, improve indigenous economies, and advance national and regional interests on the world stage'. However, Pogge (2004: 158–159) counters that it is easy to forget that, while donor states do provide aid, they do not seek to change the underlying structures that make these poor, vulnerable individuals dependent on aid in the first place.

The G8 represents the eight states that account for '48% of the global economy and 49% of global trade . . . and majority shareholder control over the International Monetary Fund and the World Bank' (Labonte and Schrecker 2007: 185). The states that make up G8 – United States, United Kingdom, Germany, France, Japan, Italy, Russia and Canada – have enormous international economic and political power (Schrecker and Labonte 2007: 285). In addition, the G8 also provides approximately 75% of the world's foreign aid. However, Labonte and Schrecker argue, the G8 is responsible for the failure of many developing states to meet the Millennium Development Goals (MDGs), particularly the goals that address ill health, because the G8 has consistently fallen short of their official development assistance targets promised to the United Nations in 2000 (Labonte and Shrecker 2007: 186).[7] With the impact of the global financial crisis in 2008, it seems even more certain that the G8 will not be forthcoming with the necessary funds to address ill health, and the small gains that some developing states have made in meeting the MDGs will be lost due to the impact of the economic crisis on state budgets and individual income levels (Perkins 2008; Gumbo 2009).

Generally, donor states prefer vertical programmes because these afford them a degree of control over project management by permitting them to target funding (Riddell 2007: 89–106). In tandem with this tendency towards directly targeted donations, developed states have increasingly provided funding through means other than governments. Since the 1980s, USAID channels its funds through NGOs, not governments (Walt and Buse 2006: 670). Even the rise of public–private partnerships has been linked to the interests of rich states in involving national pharmaceutical companies and neoliberal lending organizations such as the World Bank in health care programmes that introduce user-pay health care and drug supply programmes, at the expense of measures aimed at building local capacity and sustaining effective long-term health care (Richards 2001; Fidler et al. 2003: 100–102).

In summary, donor states determine the agenda of 'global health governance' in terms of their funding priorities and thus, in turn, exert considerable influence over the type of health programmes and initiatives that are promoted in many aid-recipient states (Brown et al. 2006; Buchanan and Decamp 2006).

Aid-recipient states

It is often argued that health issues cross borders (Kickbusch 2007: 91; Fidler and Gostin 2008: 16). Whether the issue is pandemic preparedness, tobacco control or sanitation, analysts contend that state policies need to become less insular due to globalization (Yach and Bettcher 1998b; Kickbusch 2004). This raises the thorny question of whether aid-recipient states are ready to relinquish their relatively recently acquired sovereignty in the name of health threats that they have long confronted.

Much of this chapter has focused on the impact of external actors on individuals within states. From WHO to the MSF to donor states, the argument has been that global actors play an important role in shaping domestic health agendas in the field of 'global health governance'. I have highlighted the struggle among international organizations for 'power and influence' in determining health policy (Buse et al. 2002: 265). I have also shown that non-state actors are increasingly playing an important role in setting health agendas and allocating resources. Donor states have always had an important role, and this role too can be beset by political and economic interests that suit donors' needs more than the recipient states. However, '[I]t is quite true, of course, that local economic institutions, and local factors more generally, play an important role in the reproduction of extreme poverty in the developing world' (Pogge 2004: 139). Thomas Pogge argues that flawed domestic institutions and policies are partly the product of the global structures that they must exist within (2004: 139). In this final section, I explore the nature of these local institutions among aid-recipient states, and examine whether their role in 'global health governance' is at the whim of these other actors or if, indeed, their role is greater (whether good or bad) than we have so far considered.

First of all, I want to make it clear that the countries being referred to as 'aid recipient' in this section are predominantly low-income and some marginal middle-income countries (see n.2). Most of these countries have extremely poor health care systems and account for the highest number of preventable illnesses and deaths.[8] One example of the important link between poverty, equality and health is provided in the WHO 2007 health statistics report: in Mozambique, when household wealth quintiles (the quality of building construction, number of rooms, etc.) are compared between the wealthiest and the poorest – access to clean drinking water makes a 19% difference to a child's health, while the type of dwelling makes a 17% difference (WHO 2007a: 17).

Second, I use the term 'engage' to identify the fact that there is not much discussion of the role of aid-recipient states in shaping global health governance (Thomas and Weber 2004). The role of donor states and international organizations such as WHO and UNICEF, and private organizations such as the Gates Foundation, is more often referred to and examined. By contrast, there is little discussion of the role of aid-recipient states themselves in shaping the health of their citizens. Yet there are a number of difficult questions that should be examined. For example, why has the Ugandan government not yet been able to provide safe drinking water to all of its provinces in spite of extensive foreign aid in this area? In 2008, Save the Children issued a report arguing that governance practices of aid-recipient states themselves were an increasing problem, but not yet widely recognized. Consider the following examples. South Africa's President Thabo Mbeki's refusal to accept a link between HIV and AIDS did not damage his party nor cancel his invitations to G8 Summits. Sierra Leone has received increased aid and foreign investment since the end of its civil war, but there has been no measurable change to the lives of its poorest citizens. Nor is there much discussion about why the continued lack of affordable health care in Bangladesh is not a leading issue in its national elections, despite long-established links between poverty and health outcomes. In addition to these individual cases, neoliberal reforms imposed by the World Bank have allowed some politicians to get away with the sweeping claim that they have no responsibility for their citizens' health (Save the Children 2008).

Political engagement with health inequalities *within* aid-recipient states has not occurred at the level that one might expect. Fidler argues that 'developments over the last decade have forced public health experts and diplomats to think of health *as* foreign policy, namely public health as important to states' pursuit of their interests and values in international relations' (2007a: 53), which has resulted in health policy being associated with political and economic security rather than addressed in its own right, and only to some extent as a human right (see chapter 3). Although governments complain about World Bank conditionality, few affected states – if any – have reduced military spending to boost health spending (Hyatt 2007). Even in aid-dependent states where there is a relatively high level of democracy, there remains a degree of antipathy towards health as a political issue (Farmer 2005; de Waal 2006).

The impact of the global economy on the health policy of aid-recipient states tells another tale of differing perceptions and realities. Improving primary health care provisions so that citizens have access to basic health care services would require an increase of approximately five times the current health care spending in aid-recipient countries (People's Health Movement et al. 2005: 59). The reasons for the generally low levels of health spending in many low-income and some middle-income countries include the worldwide recessions in the mid-1970s and 1980s that led to a decline of exports, interest rate increases on foreign loans, and structural adjustment programmes for health care, reducing the cash available for health spending (Koivusalo and Ollila 1997). Since the 2002 transition from SAPs to PRSPs, when the Millennium Development Goals were attached to poverty reduction plans, there has been little progress towards increasing health spending. Jeffrey Sachs describes the IMF and World Bank as having 'split personalities, championing the MDGs in public speeches, approving programmes that will not achieve them and privately acknowledging, with business as usual, that they cannot be met!' (quoted in Wamala et al. 2007: 247). Yet, as discussed above, at the micro level within many countries political neglect of citizens' basic health care needs is evident in the prioritization of military expenditure and corrupt practices that often helped cripple the few health care provisions that existed (Hyatt 2007a). The question is whether this failure is the product of state-led decision making, the global failure to develop corporate rules prohibiting corrupt practices, or whether blame should be equally shared by both the national and international actors (Pogge 2002: 21–22).

In summary, aid-recipient states are constrained to some extent by external global actors such as donor states, international organizations, even NGOs and philanthropic foundations. However, these external influences do not reduce the overall effect that these state governments could have on the health of their citizens. As revealed in this section, these same states still choose to prioritize military expenditure over health expenditure and corrupt practices over health expenditure, and cultural arguments may be put forward as arguments to deny health practices or ban health education (see chapter 3). Therefore, though there is an increased focus on actors that work on the 'global' stage of health governance, aid-recipient states still have important choices to make – which are not restrained by global actors or the global system – to take responsibility for their populations' health.

Conclusion

The preamble to the 1946 WHO Constitution states that 'Governments have a responsibility for the health of their peoples which can be fulfilled only by the provision of adequate health and social measures' (WHA 2006). As shown in this chapter, the primary responsibility of the state in the area of public health has been diluted to some extent by the emergence of actors such as international organizations, NGOs and philanthropic foundations. There has been a shift from the state as the sole actor able to singularly change the health status of an individual and the state as the sole actor that co-operates with other states on international health policy, to a context where there are very different types of actors, each with their own agendas in specific areas of public health policy.

Buse et al. (2002: 270) argue that international health becomes global health when the 'causes or consequences of a health issue circumvent, undermine or are oblivious to the territorial boundaries of states and, thus, beyond the capacity of states to address effectively through state institutions alone'. However, as demonstrated in this chapter, it is not just the health issues themselves that represent the arrival of 'global health' but also the evolution of global actors that are able to affect health policy decisions made at the state level. What is yet to be established, as Fidler (2007) asks, is whether the proliferation of so many actors shaping the political decisions that concern public health actually corresponds with increased health care response capacity and better health outcomes? I contend that, as the final section revealed, the state remains the dependent variable. In particular, the implicit assumption that aid-recipient states are powerless in the face of global health governance because they have not been provided with sufficient economic and political support from donor states, international organizations, NGOs and now PPPs does not hold up to scrutiny (de Waal 2006). This does not, however, remove donor states, NGOs and philanthropic organizations from the equation. These actors have an increasingly influential impact on local health outcomes. In the following chapters, I will demonstrate how the tension between the responsibility of the state, the health needs of individuals and the increased impact of global actors underpins responses to a range of different health issues.

3 HEALTH AS A HUMAN RIGHT

In chapter 1, we noted that the globalist perspective promotes a human rights framework as one solution to the neglect by states of their citizens' health needs. Globalists argue that, in order to prioritize the health of individuals, their right to health may be a solution to the tendency of some states to ignore their citizens' health needs. If a right to health is grounded in law and policy, it would be harder for states to avoid their responsibility. On the other hand, statists may not disagree with the utility of the right to health, but would argue that such a claim still requires state recognition and implementation of structures that can meet this right. Furthermore, how the right should be defined and fulfilled will be open to differing state interpretation. As a result, health as a human right has not achieved the same 'high politics' status in international policy circles as, say, pandemic preparedness. In chapter 2, I argued that global health governance comprises a plethora of actors that jostle and compete for funding and influence. Building on these insights, this chapter examines the 'health as a human right' movement and argues that while the right to health is a well-established aspiration there is little clarity about what it entails, which actors are responsible for satisfying it, and how.

This chapter proceeds in four parts. In the first section, I will trace how health as a human right first came to be articulated in relation to the theory of rights. The second section will then trace the emergence of the 'health as a human right' movement in the 1980s.[1] This movement developed as a strategy to win the hearts and minds of donor states, aid-recipient states and international organizations (who were often also involved in the movement) by referring to health care and treatment as a right that individuals could claim and which states had a duty to respect, protect and fulfil.

However, as the second section will argue, advocates have struggled to translate rights language into a form of politics that rewarded states for making improvements to health care systems. This is largely because the focus has remained on the right to access health care rather than the instrumental question of who should provide and fund health care. These problems are most pronounced in the attempts to secure treatment and non-discrimination for those infected with HIV/AIDS and in the movement to empower women seeking access to reproductive health care (Gruskin et al. 2007: 449), discussed (respectively) in the third and fourth sections of the chapter.

Development of health as a human right

> The enjoyment of the highest attainable standard of health is one of the fundamental rights of every human being without distinction of race, religion, political belief, economic or social condition. (WHO Constitution: WHA 2006: 1)

The World Health Organization (WHO) Constitution (1948) states that health is a universal right. In so doing, the WHO Constitution defined health as 'a state of complete physical, mental and social well-being' (WHA 2006: 1). The association between health and human rights has been reaffirmed since the establishment of WHO. It was enshrined, for instance, in the 1948 Universal Declaration of Human Rights which stated that:

1. Everyone has the right to a standard of living adequate for the health and well-being of himself and of his family, including food, clothing, housing and medical care and necessary social services, and the right to security in the event of unemployment, sickness, disability, widowhood, old age or other lack of livelihood in circumstances beyond his control.
2. Motherhood and childhood are entitled to special care and assistance. All children, whether born in or out of wedlock, shall enjoy the same social protection. (Article 25, UNGA 1948)

Moreover, the 1966 International Covenant on Economic, Social and Cultural Rights (ICESCR), which came into force in 1976, expressed the right to health in the following way:

1. The State Parties to the present Covenant recognize the right of everyone to the enjoyment of the highest attainable standard of physical and mental health.

2. The steps to be taken by the State Parties to the present Covenant to achieve the full realization of this right shall include those necessary for:
    (a) The provision for the reduction of the stillbirth rate and of infant mortality and for the healthy development of the child;
    (b) The improvement of all aspects of environmental and industrial hygiene;
    (c) The prevention, treatment and control of epidemic, endemic, occupational and other diseases;
    (d) The creation of conditions which would assure to all medical service and medical attention in the event of sickness. (Article 12, UNGA 1966)

It is worth noting that none of these articles provides indicators for when the right to health has been fulfilled (Toebes 1999a). Whether the identification of such responsibilities is possible is, in some part, key to realizing the 'right to health'. Critics argue that the right to health is impossible to achieve because it either implies that there is such a thing as perfect health or that individuals need no more than the right conditions for good health to prevail. This denies, of course, that an individual's genetic predisposition to disease, disability and infirmity and an individual's own lifestyle choices are also important factors (Aginam 2005a: 5). It also denies the possibility that the provision of other sorts of rights, such as social and economic freedoms, can improve individual health (Mann et al. 1999).

Access and provision

At the heart of the debate about health and human rights is a tension between access and provision that mirrors the philosophical distinction between negative and positive rights. Simply put, negative rights require that actors refrain from certain types of activity that infringe on the rights of others. For instance, the right to life, the right to be free from torture, and the right to choose one's religion only require that actors desist from killing people, torturing them and inhibiting their freedom to choose their religion. In their simplest form, they do not require positive action to ensure their fulfilment. By contrast, positive rights are rights that require actors to take positive steps to ensure their fulfilment. Positive rights require that the state make social, economic and legislative changes to accommodate and provide these rights. The right to education, the right to shelter and the right to clean water are positive rights because they require duty-bearers to make material provisions to provide them, rather than simply refrain from certain courses of action. Jack Donnelly describes the difference between them as being that negative rights only requires the 'forbearance on the part of others', while positive rights requires 'others to provide goods, services, or opportunities' (2003: 30). However, critics contend that the bifurcation of rights into negative and positive rights is of little moral significance because even negative rights require positive duties for their fulfilment. For instance, the ban on smoking indoors requires that someone police it. Likewise, Donnelly argues that 'all human rights required both positive action and restraint on the part of the state' (2003: 30). Therefore, the idea that any right requires no actual material change to the behaviour of actors has been largely debunked.

Despite this view, the distinction between negative and positive rights has been important in the debate about health as a human right. There is a big difference between the insistence that 'all I have to do is not prevent people seeking the best health care they can afford', which is a negative right based on the 'do no harm principle', and a claim that 'I have a duty to ensure that every person is able to access the best health care possible', which is implied by the positive rights approach. The distinction in understanding what a human right to health means is one between *access* (the right to seek care and not be prevented from doing so with no specific duty-bearer assuming responsibility for the provision of care) and *provision* (the right to be provided with the best care possible with a duty-bearer having an obligation to ensure that such provision is made available). This distinction is important for understanding the 'empirical circumstances' (Donnelly 2003: 31) surrounding how the right to health is claimed and fulfilled as well as the scope of the right itself.

In the area of health, the tension between access – the obligation not to deny access to basic health care – and provision – the obligation to provide basic health care to all – pivots around two key questions. First, what is the scope of the right and responsibility to fulfil this right in relation to access and provision? Second, on whom does the obligation fall? In the main, the health and human rights movement has argued that the responsibility is shared between those seeking better health (i.e. the individual), those who have the power to deny or allow access (i.e. the state), and those who see inequality in the provision of the right as it is at present and seek to plug the gaps (i.e. the international donor community, including NGOs) (Hunt 2003; Gruskin et al. 2005). However, in practice the scope and focus of responsibility remains hotly contested, limiting the ability of rights language to deliver tangible improvements in the provision of health care.

The 'health as a human right' movement

As noted earlier, the link between health and human rights was established by WHO's mandate and has been unanimously endorsed by states since then. No government argued, for example, that health should not constitute a right during the drafting of the WHO Constitution, the Universal Declaration of Human Rights or the International Covenant on Economic, Social and Cultural Rights (Toebes 1999a). However, neither was it clear *whose* responsibility it was to realize this right, *how* the right would be realized and *when* the right to health had been satisfied (Taylor 1992: 327). As Tomasevski argued, 'public health spelled out individual obligations rather than rights' (2005: 3). Emphasis was placed mostly on what the individual should do to improve their health. According to Paul Hunt, the UN's special rapporteur on the right to health (appointed in 2002), the 'right to health' remained 'little more than a slogan for more than 50 years' (2007: 369). It was not, he maintained, until the UN Committee on Economic, Social and Cultural Rights adopted General Comment 14 in 2000 that it became clearer what the right to health encompassed. The General Comment confirmed that:

> [T]he express wording of article 12.2 acknowledges that the right to health embraces a wide range of socio-economic factors that promote conditions in which people can lead a healthy life, and extends to the underlying determinants of health, such as food and nutrition, housing, access to safe and potable water and adequate sanitation, safe and healthy working conditions, and a healthy environment. . . [5.] The Committee is aware that, for millions of people throughout the world, the full enjoyment of the right to health still remains a distant goal. Moreover, in many cases, especially for those living in poverty, this goal is becoming increasingly remote. The Committee recognizes the formidable structural and other obstacles resulting from international and other factors beyond the control of States that impede the full realization of article 12 in many States parties. [6.] With a view to assisting States parties' implementation of the Covenant and the fulfilment of their reporting obligations, this General Comment focuses on the normative content of article 12 (Part I), States parties' obligations (Part II), violations (Part III) and implementation at the national level (Part IV), while the obligations of actors other than States parties are addressed in Part V. (UN Committee on Economic, Social and Cultural Rights 2000)

The problem that remained even after General Comment 14 has been getting states to agree to the aspects of the right to health requiring simple access from the state – for example, freedom from discrimination – and aspects requiring the positive provision of goods by the state.

Arguably, WHO has an international mandate to draft legal conventions that would define the rights and responsibilities of all actors more clearly (Gruskin et al. 2007: 450). However, budgetary pressures from the United States and other donors (see chapter 2), an internal reluctance to use international law to enforce its mandate, and confusion about whose health such rights were to protect, prompted WHO to shy away from advancing legal responsibilities in relation to the right to health (Taylor 1992). For example, the 'right to health' was expressed in the 1978 WHO-UNICEF-led Alma Ata Declaration on Primary Health Care, and again in the 1986 Ottawa Charter, but the 'unacceptable' inequalities of health care that both declarations proclaimed did not lead to specific guidelines or even a shared understanding of what should be done about the provision of public health (Thomas and Weber 2004; Manciaux and Fliedner 2005).

The effort to actualize the right to health was therefore spearheaded by key individuals such as Jonathan Mann, who with Lawrence Gostin, Sofia Gruskin, Troyen Brennan, Zita Lazzarini and Harvey Fineberg pioneered a three-part framework for linking health and human rights. Mann and his colleagues focused on the link between health and other pre-existing social, political and economic rights. As head of the WHO's Global Programme of Action on HIV/AIDS (1987–1996, disbanded to create UNAIDS), Mann's principal aim was to raise the profile of HIV/AIDS as a human rights issue. However, Mann et al. made a wider contribution by demonstrating the link between persistent socio-economic inequalities and health outcomes. First, they argued that public health programmes should be treated as potential burdens, even violations, of human rights until proven otherwise. For example, limitations on the 'rights of the few' for the 'good of the many' had often been used as a justification for infectious disease control, mandatory testing and treatment, as well as isolation (Mann et al. 1999: 13). As a result, every time that a public health decision restricts or ignores human rights the 'prevailing assumption that public health . . . is an unalloyed public good that does not require consideration of human rights norms' (Mann et al. 1999: 13) takes shape as a normal part of public health policy, and therefore becomes harder to challenge. Second, human rights violations always have an impact on health, be it torture, withholding valid health information or withholding treatment. Third, health as a human right should take a complementary approach that understands health as the realization of three factors: physical, mental and social well-being. Linking health to human rights was therefore the best mechanism for individuals to attain their best personal outcomes in these three areas. According to Mann, how an individual was diagnosed, what treatment they had access to and what conditions led to them contracting the disease all had human rights implications (Mann in Gostin and Lazzarini 1997: 169).

Naturally, advocates agreed with Mann's proposition that health as a human right required change to social, economic and political structures in order to ensure equality, access and distributive justice (Mann 1999; Pogge 2004; Gruskin and Tarantola 2005). Where they differed was in emphasis and priorities. Was the right to health something sought through access to other rights (right to education, equality, freedom of speech, non-discrimination), or is there some free-standing right to health that imposes obligations on duty-bearers that is distinct from other rights? Mann, who was seeking to raise the profile of HIV/AIDS as a human rights issue, argued that in the case of AIDS the 'vulnerability of people to these health problems seemed integrally connected to the status of realization of their human rights' (Mann in Gostin and Lazzarini 1997: 168). In other words, he maintained that the right to health was ultimately dependent on the provision of other human rights such as non-discrimination and privacy. Paul Farmer does not disagree with Mann, but he has also argued that health as a human right may require the imposition of positive duties in its own right, such as access to medical care being construed as equivalent to the right to vote (2005: 238–246). The question is, are these two positions mutually exclusive or not: can health be a positive right and be linked to other rights? The answer depends on who is responsible to realize the right to health.

The ICESCR's Article 12 states that the right to health requires states to recognize the right of everyone to the enjoyment of the highest attainable standard of physical and mental health. The UN's Paul Hunt argues that this means that states have an obligation to *respect, protect* and *fulfil* the right to health, as mentioned in General Comment 14 (see above). However, there are three potential problems with this conceptualization of state obligation. First, the right to physical and mental health implies that states will provide the necessary means for individuals to access health care (Toebes 1999b). However, the obligation to pursue the right to health remains a general principle rather than a specific one (Tomasevski 2005), as we will see in the discussion on HIV/AIDS and reproductive health, below. As a result, there is no specific obligation to ensure that individuals attain physical and mental health and no guidelines for how the state's obligations are to be discharged. Second, the distributive obligation in the area of public health and the extent of each state's legal responsibility to each individual is far from clear (Taylor 1992; Yamin 1996; Thomas and Weber 2004). For example, the Constitutional Court of South Africa ruled in 2002 that all newborns and their HIV-infected mothers were entitled to the antiretroviral drug, nevirapine, to prevent HIV transmission from mother to child. However, the Court's determination that a treatment such as nevirapine should be available to all HIV-infected mothers has not translated into the government ensuring that there is the money and staff available to provide this treatment to all women who need it in South Africa (Dorrington et al. 2006: 14–15). In the UK, the courts have traditionally avoided making judgements around the state provision of health care because 'difficult and agonizing judgements have to be made as to how a limited budget is best allocated to the maximum advantage of maximum number of patients. This is not a judgement which the court can make' (emphasis added, R. v Cambridge Health Authority [1995]). Finally, the right to health has not created a corresponding duty to refrain from impairing a state's responsibility to satisfy its (health) obligations. While the World Trade Organization (WTO) Doha Declaration on the Trade Related Aspects of Intellectual Property Rights Agreements (TRIPS) affirmed its members' right to protect public health, access to affordable pharmaceuticals was blocked by the requirement that the drug in question only have its patent removed if the state proved that the disease in question was of *epidemic* and *emergency* proportions. In this case, the right to access reasonably priced generic drugs because no individual should die for lack of readily available treatment – which would seem to derive from the right to health – did not trump the commercial rights of pharmaceutical companies (see chapter 7).

It is clear, therefore, that the obligations set out under the ICESCR are not legally binding and their application is unclear. Furthermore, only sixty-two states have ratified the ICESCR into their domestic legislation, making it difficult to use it as a benchmark for ascertaining the scope of states' responsibility to deliver on the right to health. Advocates such as Sofia Gruskin (2004: 320) argue that, by virtue of a state signing on to ICESCR, the Convention against the Elimination of Discrimination Against Women (CEDAW) and the Convention on the Rights of the Child (CROC), and even the Doha Declaration on TRIPS, they have accepted an *implicit* obligation to improve health and establish health as a human right. However, careful reading of the ICESCR reveals that signatory states only have such obligations if they have the capacity (as measured by the state itself) to provide the required measures and even then the extent to which the state must respect, protect and fulfil these rights is not clearly defined (UNESCR 2000). The state's 'obligation' to meet the health needs of its citizens is not institutionalized and there are no clear political consequences for non-compliance. Institutionalization is important in this regard, because it is through institutionalization that rights language is translated into pressure to change behaviour (Risse and Sikkink 1999: 33). In addition, there has been little agreement about the practical demands levied by health as a human right, which human rights norms should be institutional-ized, and which institutions are the appropriate duty-bearers.

This section has shown that there have been advances in the articulation of health as human right through various international legal instruments and advocacy by Jonathan Mann and others who sought to demonstrate that health is a human right and is fulfilled when it is integrated into the broader matrix of socio-economic rights. However, there has been little change in actual behaviour among the actors who could best institutional-ize the right to health, particularly in the case of HIV/AIDS and women's health, discussed below. Nor has the lack of progress to deliver on their commitments been regarded as a failure on the part of states (Thomas 2000; Aginam 2005a; Farmer 2005). The challenges that arise from this are clearly apparent in connection with international efforts to promote the HIV/AIDS human rights movement and the reproductive rights movement.

HIV/AIDS and human rights

In 1981, a disease was identified among homosexual males in San Francisco (Beaglehole and Bonita 2004: 86–87). The disease had a dev-astating effect on the immune system and was passed not just through sexual activity, but also via blood transfusions, shared needles, giving birth and breast feeding. Within twenty-six years, the human immunodeficiency virus/acquired immune deficiency syndrome (HIV/AIDS) had infected 33.2 million people (range 30.6–36.1 million), including 2.5 million chil-dren under the age of fifteen (UNAIDS 2007: 3, 8). Because the disease was first associated with homosexual activity and then with unprotected sexual activity in general, there was widespread discrimination against those who were diagnosed with HIV (Kallings 2008). When little was known about the disease, it was not uncommon for hospitals to refuse treatment to infected patients for fear of cross-infection. Some govern-ments and religious organizations denied that the disease existed, or used the disease to discriminate against those infected, sometimes even arresting infected individuals. At the same time, the cultural stigma surrounding HIV/AIDS within countries such as China, India and South Africa led to under-reporting (Annas 1999a; Poku 2005; Kallings 2008). The prolonged silence by governments contributed to misinformation pertaining on how HIV led to AIDS and, most crucially, a lack of education campaigns to prevent the spread of infection.

Jonathan Mann argued that 'in each society, those people who before HIV/AIDS arrived were marginalized, stigmatized and discriminated against became over time those at highest risk of HIV infection' (1999: 221). The fact that HIV mainly targeted those who were already poor and disenfranchised meant that potential victims were all the more vulnerable to misinformation and stigma, which was why articulating their right to education, care and treatment was all the more vital (Mann 1999). Misinformation was allowed to spread because of the time lag between HIV infection and AIDS illness, sometimes eight to ten years, which contributed to the perception – voiced by some prominent figures such as South African President Thabo Mbeki – that there was no link between HIV and AIDS (de Waal 2006: 12). This encouraged governments to avoid investment in testing and preventive measures. Denial was a big problem in the 1980s and arguably remains a key obstacle to AIDS awareness to this day (Poku 2005: 4). Mann argued that misinformation was allowed to continue so long in the case of AIDS because those most vulnerable to the disease – women, gay men, drug users and children – were also disempowered and denied other basic political and social rights (Mann 1999: 214).

That little care was provided to those infected with HIV was also rooted in the fact that those most at risk of the disease, especially in Asia and Africa, inhabited regions with competing major health problems such as tuberculosis, malaria and diarrhoeal disease (Kallings 2008: 235). Nor should the political and cultural problems with AIDS awareness and treatment be discounted. Depending on culture and religion, admitting to prostitution, drug abuse or homosexuality could lead to social isolation and discrimination; particular states and particular religious institutions (e.g. Islam and the Roman Catholic church) were reluctant or just refused to acknowledge the need to discuss safe sex for homosexual and heterosexual relationships (Kallings 2008: 235). As a result, the time lag between raising awareness and preventing harmful infectious behaviour (or providing safe mechanisms for prostitutes, drug users and people with multiple sexual partners) led to the 1980s being a decade of lost potential in combating the disease (Lewis 2005).

Because of the nature of primary HIV infection – either through drug use or sexual behaviour (the exception is children who are born to HIV-positive mothers) – there was always going to be contestation over whose role it was to raise awareness about HIV/AIDS, and whose responsibility it was to test for HIV, and best manage treatment of those with the disease (Lewis 2005). The nature of HIV/AIDS meant that it could not be treated like any other infectious disease emergency (De Cock and Johnson 1998). For example, testing is difficult because HIV can lie dormant for up to 18 months after initial infection, which means that people have to undergo regular testing. In addition, AIDS can lie dormant for years, which means that people may not be diagnosed with HIV until they are gravely ill with AIDS. These particulars of HIV make it easier for individuals to inadvertently spread the disease. Moreover, the little that was known about HIV/AIDS allowed many myths and fears to dominate public perceptions. One result was that many hid their diagnosis, putting others at risk, or died early through failing to seek treatment. Finally, the association between homosexual behaviour and the HIV/AIDS pandemic encouraged governments to respond by introducing or reinforcing anti-sodomy laws. The result of this was imprisonment and in some cases torture of homosexual men, accusations of homosexuality levelled against political opponents, and increased vulnerability of women and children who were sometimes wrongly portrayed as immune from the disease (Gostin and Lazzarini 1997; Mann and Tarantola 1998; Farmer 2005; de Waal 2006).

In response, Jonathan Mann and other UN officials, human rights activists, gay activists, individual carers and victims started to campaign against the various forms of discrimination being practised against HIV/AIDS victims (Gostin and Lazzarini 1997; Gostin and Mann 1999). In the late 1980s, officials from WHO and UNICEF campaigned with individuals in USA and Europe, then Africa and Asia, against quarantine measures, separate treatment clinics and legislative attempts to revoke the slender advances in gay rights that had been achieved during the 1970s (mostly in the United States and Europe). At the same time, this movement stressed the right of individuals to have access to health care that focused on detection, treatment and prevention of HIV/AIDS.

The breakthrough was Mann's argument that the detection, treatment and prevention of HIV/AIDS could not be treated as 'just' a health concern, but that it also had to be dealt with as a human rights issue (Gostin and Lazzini 1997; Gruskin 2004; de Waal 2006). Mann identified three periods of HIV prevention efforts, tracing how the human rights approach emerged. The first stage between 1981 and 1984 involved, essentially, scare tactics. 'Don't die of Ignorance' was a banner associated with AIDS awareness. The messages did not resolve myths about HIV infection. Fear only heightened discrimination, so between 1985 and 1988, awareness changed with the focus shifting to individual risk reduction. During the same period, in 1987, WHO's Special Program on AIDS (later named the Global Program on AIDS [GPA]) was adopted by the UN General Assembly. Mann, who was director of the GPA, argued that the Program led an 'unprecedented' global AIDS strategy (Mann 1999: 217). The coercion and discrimination that WHO officials witnessed being expressed towards those infected with HIV/AIDS in both developed and developing states inspired a 'public health rationale' for preventing discrimination (Mann 1999: 217). Preventing discrimination became a stronger theme in the third stage as the global epidemic intensified after 1988 and started to affect a wider demographic in poor regions where knowledge of the disease and responses to it were minimal at best. As the disease spread throughout Africa during this period, particularly in sub-Saharan Africa, alarm bells started to ring in the halls of the UN and WHO (Mann 1999).

The global demographic spread of the disease, Mann argued, demonstrated that the major determinants of HIV/AIDS were societal (Mann 1999: 222). HIV/AIDS was the product of unprotected sex, inadequate education about the sexual transmission of the disease, shared needles and transmission through birth. The people who were most vulnerable were the poor, disenfranchised and minority groups, and their marginalization produced a 'lack of clear political commitment to take the radical steps necessary to save lives' (Kirby 1996: 1217). Therefore the GPA aimed its efforts at these groups, focusing on discrimination, promoting education about the disease, and advocating the right to confidentiality so that people would be more willing to be tested.

However, raising awareness of the disease, the right to be tested and the right to confidentiality had to be balanced against what some governments argued was their right to quarantine the infected, in order to safeguard the protection of the wider community by imprisoning those who were discovered to be infected with HIV. Moreover, some domestic environments, particularly those suspicious or hostile to the awareness campaigns required to prevent HIV in sub-Saharan Africa and the Middle East, refused particular programmes. Preventive methods such as the use of condoms, and education awareness campaigns for homosexuals, were resisted in many countries due to religious and cultural customs (Annas 1999a; Tomasevski 2005).

Therefore, incorporating human rights into HIV/AIDS prevention required the identification of 'the specific rights whose violation contributes to HIV vulnerability in one particular community or country' (Mann 1999: 223). The right to information, equality for men and women, the right to medical care and the right to non-discrimination continued as part of the HIV/AIDS prevention campaign during the 1990s. However, these campaigns experienced more success when they focused, for instance, on preventive measures such as blood screening rather than on condom distribution (Lee and Zwi 2003: 25). In addition, institutional competition between WHO, UNFPA (United Nations Population Fund) and UNICEF for AIDS funds, and disagreement among donor countries over which campaigns should receive more funding than others, led to the creation of the Joint Program on HIV/AIDS (UNAIDS) in 1996 (Lee and Zwi 2003: 25–26). UNAIDS now co-ordinates the work of ten UN agencies working on HIV/AIDS-related activities,[2] but there is no regular budget for any of its own initiatives and thus it relies on voluntary donations to fund such projects. As a result, UNAIDS has a modest annual budget of $60 million, a staff of approximately 130 headed by an executive director who is appointed by the UN Secretary-General, and most of its administrative support comes from WHO (Boone and Batsell 2007: 26; Kallings 2008: 235–236). In 2001, UN Secretary-General Kofi Annan campaigned heavily to increase UNAIDS funding through the Global Fund for AIDS, Tuberculosis and Malaria (Traub 2006: 154–155; Boone and Batsell 2007: 26). However, the $7–10 billion injection of funds required from donor countries to achieve effective treatment for these three diseases has not yet been achieved (see also chapter 2).

In the area of HIV/AIDS, the link between health and human rights has had mixed results (Siegel 1996; Harris and Siplon 2001). Take for example the debates since the late 1990s surrounding access to antiretroviral drug treatment, which can contain the side effects and development of AIDS. This has been an ongoing struggle between UNAIDS, WHO, the Global Fund to Fight AIDS, Tuberculosis and Malaria and non-governmental organizations (Schwartlander et al. 2006). The struggle is with pharmaceutical companies and whether they should allow the generic (cheaper) antiretrovirals to be produced and made available to those unable to afford the high-priced patented proprietary product. According to the WTO's TRIPS Agreement, which details the conditions in which the trade and production of patented drugs (such as antiretrovirals) can occur, only in the case of a health emergency may a country seek permission to release the patent on a particular drug so that it can be produced generically. As will be discussed in chapter 7, this has resulted in debate among actors in the 'global health governance' system as to whether such restrictions for life-saving drugs should be permissible when millions are infected and going to die from HIV/AIDS.

However, others argue that progress has been made by linking HIV/AIDS and human rights. It was the link between human security, human rights and HIV/AIDS that led to it being the first health issue taken up by the UN Security Council. The Security Council Resolution 1308 (2001) declared that AIDS posed a threat to security due to its potential devastation on humanity (Schwartlander et al. 2006: 543; for criticism see David 2001). Yet, as discussed in chapter 1, the Security Council Resolution could be seen as more a triumph for securitized approaches to health than for the 'health as a human right' movement. However, the creation of UNAIDS, a single UN agency to deal with AIDS through a universal diagnosis, treatment and prevention agenda, not to mention the repeated commitment by all UN member states to scale up their prevention, treatment, care *and* support for HIV/AIDS patients (such as the General

Assembly Special Sessions on AIDS in June 2001), demonstrates that this is at least one public health issue that has been accepted as worthy of discussion at the 'high' level of international politics. But, as demonstrated by donors' failure to invest the necessary funds into the Global Fund on AIDS, Tuberculosis and Malaria, rhetoric does not always match the reality and progress, when it can be made, is painfully slow.

The HIV/AIDS case demonstrates that efforts to link health and human rights can be crucial for saving lives. When an individual cannot be tested for HIV without fear of being imprisoned, when women continually show the highest rate of infection and when people are rejected for migrant or refugee visas due to their HIV status, we see how vital human rights are for the pursuit of good health and human well-being. However, what this case also reveals is how far we are from fulfilling the right to health. In the late 1990s, HIV/AIDS was still described by Mann and others as a disease that continued to affect those who were most vulnerable – the poor, disenfranchised and minority groups. Today, little has changed. Women are still at greatest risk of infection, particularly women of child-bearing age and living in the low socio-economic bracket (MacNaughton 2004; Kallings 2008). The regions most affected by HIV/AIDS also contain the world's poorest populations: sub-Saharan Africa, South Asia, Latin America and Central Asia (UNAIDS 2007: 8).

Emphasizing rights as part of the response to HIV/AIDS prevention and treatment has been crucial for activating a global conscience that sought to help rather than punish those infected. However, as Farmer notes, 'we have a long way to go in the struggle for health and human rights' (2005: 237). We still see that those most at risk are those least able to claim the right to services and goods that would prevent HIV infection in the first place, or ensure treatment in the early stages of the disease (Farmer 2005: 234–235). As discussed next in the case of reproductive rights, claiming the right to substantive change and ensuring the change occurs is one of the most difficult challenges for the health and human rights movement.

Reproductive rights

I have argued that to realize a human right to health we must keep in mind that there are at least two distinct needs – access and provision. There must be an obligation on behalf of a duty-bearer not to deny access to basic health care, and at the same time, an obligation to provide the best care possible. What consideration has been given then to the specific health needs of women? As this section will argue, women's right to health has taken a journey similar to the 'health as a human right' movement in general. Though there has been much effort at the international level to establish women's right to access gender-responsive health care policies, there has been little progress in ensuring that women are actually provided with gender-responsive health care policies. The problem of provision and building political pressure on states to fulfil women's health needs, like HIV/AIDS, is partly to do with the broader failure to articulate the precise scope of states' obligations. In addition, and this is specific to women's right to health, issues of forced marriage, access to contraceptives, choice surrounding unwanted pregnancies and female genital mutilation are core rights-related issues that must be dealt with in order to provide women with the best provision of health care. However, as will be shown, these issues are politically and culturally controversial, stymieing efforts to advance women's health. Moreover, the lack of consistent funding to improve women's access to health care further hinders efforts to satisfy women's health needs.

We can see the need to link health and human rights for women just from looking at the statistics. For example, in 2007 women accounted for 61% of HIV infections in sub-Saharan Africa. In Latin America, Asia and Eastern Europe the proportion of women becoming HIV-infected is increasing (UNAIDS 2007). Less than half of all women in Asia and Africa are assisted by health care personnel during birth, and 14 million adolescent girls give birth every year (UNGA 2008: 4–5).[3] Women in sub-Saharan Africa and South Asia have a lifetime risk of maternal death that is 1,000 times greater than that in industrialized regions (ibid.). The likelihood of achieving the fifth Millennium Development Goal, which calls for a three-quarters reduction in maternal-related deaths by 2015, is remote. Indeed, between 1990 and 2005, there were 535,900 maternal deaths each year and the numbers in sub-Saharan Africa and South Asia show little sign of improvement (Hill et al. 2007). Between 1995 and 2003, 48% of all abortions were unsafe, causing at least half a million deaths each year (Sedgh et al. 2007: 1344).

Today, those fighting for improvements to women's reproductive health refer to these statistics as proof that women's right to decide on matters relating to their sexual health, and access to health treatment in general, is pivotal (Glasier et al. 2006; Low et al. 2006). However, in line with the general 'health as a human right' movement, the reproductive health movement has approached from different perspectives what rights women need in order to control and improve their health. *Right to reproductive self-determination* advocates argue that women do not just need family planning services, they also need the autonomy to decide when they should have sex and with whom, and a choice of reproductive health care options (Cook et al. 2003; Kelly and Cook 2007; Asal et al. 2008). The self-determination movement maintains that the right to refuse sex and the right to contraceptive choice have to inform a major part of a woman's right to health (Tomasevski 2005: 7). By contrast, *right to reproductive health care* advocates argue that women need to enjoy access to safe, high-quality reproductive and sexual health care first. In particular, they argue that the right of self-determination is more an 'end product' than one which is necessary for the fulfilment of other rights (Cottingham and Myntti 2002: 83–109; Menken and Rahman 2005: 96–98). The right to reproductive health care movement argues that the provision of services such as access to basic health care and reproductive services may in fact be more important than the right to sexual and reproductive self-determination. Socio-political rights such as the right to choose contraceptive devices and access to particular services, the right to refuse sex, and the right to public sex education are all important, but they will follow once health care is promoted as the first and foremost priority (Low et al. 2006).

The difference between the two camps on which reproductive right should come first is reflected in the articulation of reproductive rights through responses to HIV/AIDS, family planning and sex education programmes.[4] States and international organizations also take different positions according to one of these views.[5] However, neither school has wavered on the need for women's health to be expressed as a *right* (Yamin 2005; Buse et al. 2006; Cleland et al. 2006). Because of this unified rights focus, I will refer to the reproductive health rights movement as a single group for the purpose of this chapter, but it is worth noting the differences between them in how they seek gains in reproductive rights for women.

The subordination of women's health has a long history. Women's lack of education has long been associated with the premature death of their children (Starrs 2007: 1285); their reproductive health has been dominated by myth, superstition and trivialization, resulting in the widespread use of local remedies, forced circumcision and social exclusion (Doyal 1995). To understand how the language of rights has been used to address some of these problems, I will briefly recount some of the international efforts. The 1979 Convention on the Elimination of Discrimination against Women (CEDAW) demanded women's right to health and was seen as a break-through because it 'explicitly addresses human rights regarding family planning services, care and nutrition during pregnancy, information, and, for instance, education to decide the number and spacing of one's children' (Cook et al. 2003: 153–154). However, its reference to health was limited to one article, Article 12, and largely discussed women's health in the context of family planning:

1. States Parties shall take all appropriate measures to eliminate discrimination against women in the field of health care in order to ensure, on a basis of equality of men and women, access to health care services, including those related to family planning.
2. Notwithstanding the provisions of paragraph I of this article, States Parties shall ensure to women appropriate services in connection with pregnancy, confinement and the post-natal period, granting free services where necessary, as well as adequate nutrition during pregnancy and lactation. (UNGA 1979)

In a similar way as the ICESCR, the CEDAW required signatory states to establish the capacity to deliver on women's right to health, but provided no political or funding incentives on how this might be achieved. Nor has there been consensus among the international women's movement that the Convention's focus on contraception best expresses the diverse health needs and lack of equity that afflict women of all age groups (Lush and Campbell 2001: 185).

The next element of the campaign to establish women's health as a human right focused on promoting women's rights through the global Safe Motherhood Initiative. The Initiative was launched in 1987 by a group of NGOs, international organizations and governments and it sought to address the health needs of mothers. The intention of the Initiative was to 'generate political will, identify effective interventions, and mobilize resources' that would prevent the death of half a million women each year during pregnancy and childbirth (99% of the deaths were in developing countries) (Starrs 2007: 1285). A recent study found that between 1990 and 2005, while there was an overall decrease of 2.5% per year in the maternal mortality ratio, there were still 535,900 maternal deaths in 2005 and the ratios in sub-Saharan Africa showed little if any improvement (Hill et al. 2007).

Around the same time as the HIV/AIDS health human rights movement appeared on the international scene, an important step came for those advocating reproductive self-determination at the 1994 UN International Conference on Population and Development (ICPD) in Cairo, Egypt (Lush and Campbell 2001; Cottingham and Myntti 2002). The ICPD recognized a Programme of Action to protect reproductive health and sexual health as a matter of social justice best realized through human rights claims (Cook et al. 2003: 148–149). A total of 179 states agreed on the definition of reproductive health – ostensibly the health care that women would have a right to claim in these countries:

[P]eople are able to have a satisfactory and safe sex life and that they have the capability to reproduce and the freedom to decide if, when and how often to do so. Implicitly in this last condition are the right of men and women to be informed and to have access to safe, effective, affordable and acceptable methods of family planning of their choice, as well as other methods of their choice for the regulation of fertility which are not against the law.' (ICPD 1994: Programme of Action, para. 7.2)

It is important to note that the ICPD outcome, as with the Safe Motherhood Initiative, placed primary emphasis on reproductive health care, and less emphasis on sexual rights (e.g. the right to have sex that is not exploitative) (Higer 1999; Richey 2005). Resources were to be dedicated towards family planning, emergency obstetric care, and diagnosis and treatment of sexually transmitted diseases including HIV/AIDS (Fathalla et al. 2006: 2098). The programme was in marked contrast to earlier reproductive health initiatives that focused more on the need to control population size, rather than women's ability to control their own fertility (Freedman 1999b: 238). However, this change of focus prompted Catholic and Islamic participants to join forces in denouncing the Conference and the Programme of Action on religious grounds (Freedman 1999a: 164).

Unsurprisingly, perhaps, the commitments made at the ICPD have not been translated into action. There were significant shortfalls in financial contributions and in finding the political will to introduce the legislative and public health provisions that would allow women to determine their reproductive health (Ngwena 2004; Glasier et al. 2006). The cost of implementing the Programme of Action was estimated to be $17 billion by 2000 and $22 billion by 2015, which was the year the Programme of Action was to come to a close (Senanayake and Hamm 2004: 70). National governments were to contribute two-thirds of their health budget to meet this investment in women's health needs, and donor states would supplement the remaining one-third. In 1997, the UNFPA announced that annual expenditure was already well below the ICPD estimated amount required to roll out the Programme of Action by 2000. Economic distress for developing countries at the time was exacerbated by their currency losing value against the US dollar, and rapid inflation affected many states' capacity to invest the required two-thirds. This meant that '80% of the investment by less developed countries comes from China, India, Indonesia, Mexico and Iran. The remainder of the less-developed countries will, therefore, have only a few tens of cents per person from domestic budgets to support the whole of reproductive health and family planning' (Potts and Walsh 1999: 315). However, the rollout of the ICPD programme was hampered not only by aid-recipient states' inability to meet their obligations but also by donor states not delivering on their financial pledges. By the time that the programme was to roll out in 2000, the United States had invested $64 million (their target was $2.2 billion), the United Kingdom $100 million (target $380 million) and Japan $100 million despite a target of $1.4 billion (Lush and Campbell 2001: 188).

The bottom line was that there was a wide gap between global aspirations and the political and cultural interests of many states. Consider, for example, the Programme of Action's likelihood of success in Egypt when, in 1992, the WHO Regional Office in Cairo published a report stating that 'to safeguard young people against sexual misbehavior, early marriages must be encouraged' (WHO 1992: 32 in Tomasevski 2005: 7). In addition, the right to access reproductive health care was limited to cases where the state was willing to make it available and providing that none of the measures violated domestic law (e.g. abortion). This meant that states were under no obligation to grant access to abortion, for instance, if it remained illegal. As a result, there was some debate among reproductive rights advocates as to whether the ICPD had gone far enough. While some argued that the gains for women were significant, others pointed out that the constraints would limit their positive impact (Higer 1999; Knudsen 2006). Nonetheless, the ICPD was considered an important step forward for reproductive health because it reoriented 'family planning away from meeting demographic targets and towards a primary level service designed to meet the needs of individual women' (Lush and Campbell 2001: 187).

What was lacking in the aftermath of the adoption of the ICPD Programme of Action was political commitment from states to deliver on these newly proclaimed rights. For the ICPD to work, women required education, access to health care to ensure safe sex, prevent and treat sexually transmitted diseases, allow access to, and a choice of, family planning measures (including safe abortion), as well as clear laws prohibiting sexual violence and setting out a minimum age for marriage (Billson 2006). The implementation of the ICPD in individual states also required the political will to overcome cultural and religious resistance. But even where political will existed in low- to middle-income countries, significant investment by the international community was not forthcoming (Cleland et al. 2006: 1881; Fathalla et al. 2006: 2095). For example, between 1995 and 2003, donor support for family planning commodities and service delivery *fell* from $560 million to $460 million (Cleland et al. 2006: 1811). While there has been an increase in maternal and newborn health funding since then, up to $1.2 billion in 2006, roughly half of this sum continues to be apportioned to child health. The consequence of fluctuating aid income and tied aid is that it complicates 'efforts for effective planning for strategic priorities in developing countries' (UNICEF 2008: 101).

Margaret Chan, Director General of WHO, has argued that the persistent failure by the international community to invest in health systems over the past two decades explains why there has been no progress in maternal health (UN Department of Public Information 2008a). But the UN Secretary-General's report on obstetric fistula also noted that, particularly in sub-Saharan Africa and South Asia, more efforts were needed to ensure that women in poor and rural regions, particularly adolescent girls, were included in national plans to address 'underlying social, cultural and economic determinants of maternal death and disability' (UNGA 2008: 18). In sum, neglect at both the international and domestic level has contributed to women's health continuing to be a 'silent emergency' (UN Department of Public Information 2008b).

The need to address sexual health was again addressed in a 1999 review of the ICPD Programme's progress. It was reaffirmed that sexual health for all was an important goal, but a year later, the Millennium Declaration did not mention the need for a universal right to sexual and reproductive health. This was followed by the subsequent failure to adopt specific benchmarks in the area of sexual and reproductive health as a Millennium Development Goal in 2000. All of this added to concerns that states had backtracked on the reproductive health agenda (Glasier and Gulmezoglu 2007: 1550). The MDG's fifth goal – to halve maternal mortality by 2015 – further raised concerns that women's health was again being reduced to a reproductive issue and attempts to gain wider sexual freedom for women had been abandoned. However, in the same year the Committee for the ICESCR included in General Comment 14 specific references to sexual and reproductive health in paragraphs 8, 14, 20, 21 and 34. In fact, paragraph 34 stated that '[S]tates should refrain from limiting access to contraceptives and other means of maintaining sexual and reproductive health, from censoring, withholding or intentionally misrepresenting health-related information, including sexual education and information, as well as from preventing people's participation in health-related matters' (UN Committee on Economic, Social and Cultural Rights 2000).

Furthermore, to readdress the MDG neglect of reproductive health care, the 2005 UN World Summit member states attached a second target to the MDG fifth goal, known as Target B, which sought to achieve universal access to reproductive health by 2015 through monitoring progress in certain areas (see table 3.1).

Both the General Comment and the World Summit document allayed concerns somewhat, but only cautious optimism has remained. First, as

Table 3.1   Target B of Millennium Development Goal 5

Target B	*Progress indicators*
Contraceptive prevalence rate	Percentage of women aged 15–49 in union currently using contraception
Adolescent birth rate	Annual number of births to women aged 15–19 per 1,000 women in that age group
Antenatal care coverage	Percentage of women aged 15–49 attended at least once during pregnancy by skilled health personnel (doctors, nurses or midwives) and the percentage attended by any provider at least four times
Unmet need for family planning	Refers to women who are fecund and sexually active but are not using any method of contraception and report not wanting any more children or wanting to delay the birth of the next child

Source: UNICEF (2008: 20)

noted above, only fifty-six countries have actually ratified the ICESCR and, therefore, their obligation to fulfil paragraph 34 in the General Comment depends on whether the state feels bound to do so. Second, the World Summit's paragraph was a declaratory reference to sexual and reproductive health – there are no specific targets to be met and some critics argue that its inclusion was more a cynical ploy to keep voices quiet than a commitment to actually deliver on a woman's right to reproductive health (Glasier et al. 2006: 1597).

In the case of reproductive rights, therefore, we see a stark contrast between access and provision (Senanayake and Hamm 2004: 70). The right to contraception and maternal health care depend not just on women having the right to seek these goods, but also on these goods being available without restraint. For example, while the ICPD included abortion in its Programme of Action, it was conditional on the state legalizing the procedure. However, we know that 'unsafe and safe abortions correspond in large part with illegal and legal abortions, respectively' (Sedgh et al. 2007: 1343); between 1995 and 2003, the proportion of all abortions that were unsafe increased from approximately 44% to 48%, primarily in countries where seeking and performing an abortion are illegal, contributing to women's greater risk of death and long-term health consequences (ibid. 1344). The disjuncture between claiming the right and having it met highlights that, while the distinction between negative and positive rights may be untenable philosophically, it can literally mean the difference between a woman dying or living.

Jack Donnelly argues that to claim 'something' as a human right is a claim to this 'thing' as being 'needed' for a life worthy of a human being' (2003: 14). From this perspective, the health and human rights movement in the area of reproductive health has been successful. Governments may have argued about the substance, but there have been few – if any – arguments against the *need* for reproductive and sexual health care. It is generally accepted that an adequate response to reproductive health is vital for the well-being of women as well as communities, and that states have responsibility in this area, as demonstrated in the 2005 World Summit document. Even if this has not resulted in better health outcomes for women, this is an important advancement in clarifying the responsibility of states. Of course, accepting that women have a right to claim sexual and reproductive health care is not the same as actually realizing that right. It is this disconnect – between the right to access and the right to provide – that women's health, as with those suffering from HIV/AIDS, becomes imperilled by the politics of who is responsible to provide what. In the conclusion, I will briefly discuss how examining the 'health as a human right' movement is important for illustrating how the expansion of actors under the global governance system has led to greater divergence on what the right to health entails, which actors are responsible for satisfying it, and how.

Conclusion

If success is measured by political behaviour and statistical outcomes then the achievements for both the HIV/AIDS and reproductive human rights movements look modest at best. Progress in linking health and human rights has not yet reduced the needs that remain for both the individual and communities on whose behalf these rights are being claimed. Recent reports on HIV/AIDS prevalence and treatment reveal that access to treatment has fallen below the WHO's modest goal of 3 million to be treated with antiretrovirals by 2005, while the continued infection of the most socially and economically vulnerable – women and children – could have dramatic consequences on communities already affected by the disease

(Horton 2006). In other words, associating AIDS with human rights has not prevented infection nor assured treatment for those increasingly vulnerable to infection. The fact that these two groups remain most vulnerable also links closely to the lack of reproductive rights and gender equality in the areas where HIV prevalence is high (MacNaughton 2004; Tsafack Temah 2008).

The polarization of political and religious actors on women's reproductive health is as strong after the ICPD as it was beforehand (Shepard 2006: 7–8). In developing countries, young women are particularly vulnerable to HIV infection because of their engagement in sexual relations with older men for financial reasons and lack of power to insist on the use of condoms. Young women are in this position in the first place because of the political and economic constraints that limit their education, their work, their status and, ultimately, their freedom and health (MacNaughton 2004; Tsafack Temah 2008). In 2004, a joint UN report argued that national governments and the international community have not recognized the 'key role of reproductive health in underpinning sustainable development' (UNDP et al. 2004: 8).

Thomas Risse and Kathryn Sikkink talk about 'agents of change' (1999: 33–35) as crucial for human rights mobilization at the national level. Failure occurs when there is ready acceptance by international institutions and some states of declaratory prescriptions without support among donors or at the local level to adopt the measures necessary to deliver sustainable change. I argue that this is what has occurred in the case of HIV/AIDS and reproductive health. There has yet to be a clear statement of what claiming women's right to health and HIV/AIDS as rights issues encompasses without deference to the political, financial and cultural obstacles, at the local state and international levels.

Andrew Cooper and colleagues thus may be right to argue that the 'recurrent claim that health is a human right . . . still has little appeal beyond the human rights community. It has almost none for the many major power governments that do not domestically recognise a national right to health' (Cooper et al. 2007: 232). While there is little normative argument against the right of individuals to make their own health choices in order to have a life of dignity, this has led to only limited progress in domestic debates on HIV/AIDS in Africa and small increases in women's rights in the area of reproductive and sexual health. It is estimated that 'if contraception were provided to the 137 million women estimated to want contraception, but who lack access, maternal mortality could fall by an additional 25–35%' (*Lancet* 2007a: 291). Approximately 97% of the estimated 20 million annual unsafe abortions are done in low- and middle-income countries. In Kenya, for example, abortion is only legal to save a mother's life, which means that 300,000 unsafe abortions are carried out every year – accounting for 50% of maternal morality (*Lancet* 2007a: 291). Recently, the overall number of HIV infections was reduced from 38.5 to 33.2 million and was reported as a 'cause for rejoicing' and 'good news for everyone, then, donors and sufferers alike' (*Economist* 2007: 92). However, it is hard to see this as good news for the 22.5 million HIV-infected individuals living in Africa, where only 1.6 million have access to antiretroviral treatment (Horton 2006: 716; UNAIDS 2007: 5, 7).

The key, as discussed at the end of chapter 2, is to identify the agents for change in the area of health as a human right and to build evidence demonstrating the specific measures that are required to satisfy the health needs of women and individuals infected with HIV. The dilemmas that face the health and human rights movement relate to the broader tensions discussed in chapter 1. A human right to health situates the individual as the key referent but its realization requires the state. The state is required to implement the legal and political policies required that allow an individual to claim the right to health. Globalists are correct in that claiming a right to health prioritizes individual needs. However, this does not resolve the problem that rights-based claims require the state to recognize that the right exists, to understand what this means, and to provide the economic, social and political foundations necessary for claiming it.

The purpose of this chapter has not been to criticize the human rights and health movement but to better understand it and the challenges it faces from an IR perspective. From a statist perspective, it should be emphasized that the ICESR declares that the state bears the responsibility to respect, protect and fulfil these rights, but a combination of donor demands, lack of political and economic interest, and cultural considerations can dramatically affect the degree of responsibility assumed by states. A globalist perspective may not disagree that the proliferation of actors in the area of health creates confusion about the locus of responsibility, but confusion about responsibility does not diffuse the responsibility of all actors that can do something to effect change, and the global health governance system should be able to require states to realize their duty to become agents of change. The human rights and health movement has secured some important achievements, sometimes in spite of aid-recipient and donor states. However, there remain considerable areas of ambiguity relating to what a right to health entails, and despite the proliferation of non-state actors, the state is still the primary actor through which individual rights can be realized. Perhaps the key issue now is not the promotion of health as a human right, but to understand and identify the positive duties that are implied by it by multiple political actors from the local to the global level. Another area that also calls on the identification of actor responsibility when there is a tension over the duty of the actors involved is cross-border migration, which will be discussed in the next chapter.

4 CROSS-BORDER MIGRATION

'Killer Diseases Among Refugees', 'Refugee camps are the emergency departments of international public health' and 'the idea that immigrants bring with them diseases such as syphilis, malaria and tuberculosis (TB) continues to be evoked as an argument against immigration' (Toole and Waldman 1993: 604; Dyer 2002: 5; Beiser 2005: 32). These are just a sample of quotes that point to how cross-border migration is commonly portrayed. In relation to health, refugees and migrants are often portrayed as disease carriers or burdens on national health resources. In this chapter, I will argue that how migrants and refugees groups are treated by states is framed by the relationship between politics and health. In particular, there is a tension between the competing demands of securing the state, its citizens and the national interests, and securing individual migrants and respecting their human rights. This tension reflects the broader tensions between statist and globalist perspectives identified in chapter 1, and the way it plays out in practice has a direct impact on the health of individuals and communities. I argue that this tension, however, is a false one as the health of individuals, communities and states is not a zero-sum game.

The difference between a refugee and migrant has been traditionally understood as one of choice. A migrant chooses to leave one place of residence for another in search of a better life; the refugee is forced to leave due to conditions beyond their control (Malkki 1995). Such characterizations are, of course, problematic. Does a migrant who leaves her country of birth for another, to secure education and employment in a Western country so that she can improve her income to support family back home, act purely by choice? In contrast, is a refugee always one who regretfully and reluctantly leaves their home country? It may be possible that some, having experienced torture and persecution, leave their country with great relief and never seek to return. Regardless of how they might have confronted different experiences, both migrants and refugees are often treated as 'health threats' by the country they seek to enter until proven otherwise (Fassil 2000; Beiser 2005).

This chapter argues that the health of migrants and refugees has important links to political decisions about assistance to them, their treatment, and acceptance in zones of both conflict and stability. In the first section on humanitarian assistance to refugees I examine whether the proliferation of global humanitarian actors has allowed governments to abdicate their responsibility to protect their citizens' right to be safe from harm. This situation, in turn, has led to the posing of deeper moral and political questions by aid agencies: is their aid keeping populations alive or it is helping states to abdicate their responsibilities? This question reflects the deeper tension that surrounds how IR views health – around the question of prioritizing the security of the state or the security of the individual. The idea of reconciling these is rarely considered in practice, as the case studies explored in this chapter, and, indeed the whole book reveal. In the second section, I map the experience of the illegal and legal migrant crossing into high-income countries. Here, the perception of both migrants and refugees is shaped by dual notions of health threat and health burden. This perception arises from the link that has been emphasized between migrants and the spread of infectious disease in high-income countries. This link has created a tension in high-income countries between the protection of these individuals' human rights and the perceived need to protect the national community from imported diseases. The result is that, instead of reducing the disease threat by improving migrants' and refugees' health, securitized responses may actually worsen health and thereby increase the threat. Moreover, the securitization of migrants' and refugees' health may be misplaced as these groups appear to pose no higher risk as disease carriers than do imported goods and tourists returning to their home country.

First, it is important to clarify the distinction between the migrant and the refugee and understand how their experiences might differ. A refugee is defined in Article 1 of the 1951 Convention Relating to the Status of Refugees (an international legal instrument detailing the identification and treatment of refugees) as:

[A] person who owing to a well-founded fear of being persecuted for reasons of race, religion, nationality, membership of a particular social group, or political opinion, is outside the country of his nationality, and is unable to or, owing to such fear, is unwilling to avail himself of the protection of that country. (UNHCR 2007a)

For the sake of this chapter, it is important to note that, essentially, a refugee must have crossed the border of their country of origin and sought asylum in another state. In addition, this precise definition requires an individual to demonstrate a well-founded fear of persecution based on belonging to one of the persecuted groups mentioned in the above definition. The Office of the United Nations High Commissioner for Refugees (UNHCR), which oversees state accessions to the Convention and is the lead agency responsible for promoting the protection of refugees and displaced persons, acknowledges that the 1951 Convention does not accommodate people fleeing war-related conditions, such as famine and generalized violence (UNHCR 2007b: 2–4). However, the UNHCR argues that people fleeing such conditions should be *treated* as refugees as the precise source of persecution should not be decisive in determining a host country's treatment of people who have fled due to a general fear for their lives (UNHCR 2007b). In most cases, such people do not receive the legal protection of refugee status in the countries that they flee to (McGuinness 2003; Hathaway 2005). To be recognized as a refugee, asylum must be claimed in a state that is a signatory to the 1951 Convention or has domestic procedures in place to process refugees. The claim of persecution is assessed by examining the individual's story and the situation of the country that they fled. Currently, there are approximately 32.9 million displaced people (UNHCR 2007b). Of this 32.9 million 'population of concern', 9.9 million are refugees and, of these, 7.2 million reside within low-income countries, often in refugee camps or makeshift accommodation, awaiting resettlement or return and dependent on humanitarian assistance from agencies such as the UNHCR, MSF and the International Committee of the Red Cross (ICRC) (UNHCR 2007b: 5–6).

In contrast, a migrant is thought to choose to leave their country of origin for another country. The reasons why a person migrates are important because of this association with choice: a choice that the person makes to seek a life elsewhere and a choice by the receiving state to accept that person. However, as mentioned above, using 'choice' as the defining distinction between a migrant and a refugee is problematic. In reality we need to differentiate between those who choose to leave for opportunities in employment or education, and those who left to alleviate extreme poverty or to avoid civil unrest. There are therefore two prevailing models when it comes to understanding migration. The first is the voluntarist perspective (pull effect) that defines migration movement as an internal push out (due to stagnation at home) or an external pull-up (promise of greater opportunity elsewhere). The second model is the structuralist political-economy perspective (push effect), where migration is understood as a product of the global division of labour and economic wealth between the societies

in the global North and the peripheral societies of the global South (Papastergiadis 2000: 17).

In relation to health, the distinction between a migrant and a refugee is
vital. Migrants, particularly those leaving on a genuinely voluntary basis,
though still subject to medical checks, are generally welcomed to their new
country. In contrast, the forced migrant is mostly unwanted, but often
willing to take the dirty, dangerous and difficult jobs (3D jobs) that nationals are unwilling to do. Thus, they may or may not be tolerated, but their
stay will still be illegal. This type of migrant, like the refugee, often comes
from states that are weakened by political, social and economic instability.
Because health systems in their country of origin are usually of poor
quality, these individuals, not unlike refugees, may often be deemed to be
'carriers of disease' who must be monitored to ensure the safety of host
states as they will not have undergone health checks before their illegal
entry (Palinkas et al. 2003; Beiser 2005; Allotey and Zwi 2007).

We can see the tension between globalist aspirations and the statist
reality in the fact that although refugees and migrants are accorded special
rights, the inevitable distinction between desirable and undesirable migrants
and refugees can be exacerbated by perceptions of whether their health
conditions constitute a 'threat' to the state that they seek to enter. Whether
this perception is fair or accurate, it influences ideas about what counts as
'desirable' migration on the part of states. But it also creates a cyclical
problem, as will be shown below: the poorer the conditions that refugees
and illegal or undesirable migrants are forced to endure, the more likely it
is that their situation and health condition will remain or become vulnerable (Thomas 2003; Spiegel and Qassim 2003; Farmer 2005; Seal et al.
2005).

Humanitarian assistance to refugees

Conditions in most refugee camps are, to say the least, harsh. Where security is at risk, women, children and the elderly are most vulnerable. Unac-
companied women in camps can find it hard to secure shelter, adequate
food and water rations, medical care and protection from physical and
sexual violence (Djeddah 1995; Olness 1998; Allotey and Zwi 2007).
Children, who mostly rely on female care-givers, are particularly at risk
from malnutrition, as well as violence, abduction into militias and disease
due to malnourishment and poor immune defence (Toole and Waldman
1993; Olness 1998). There are dangers for men too: in refugee camps on
the Thailand–Cambodia border during the 1970s and 1980s, in Rwandan
camps in Zaire (Democratic Republic of Congo) and in Afghan camps on

the Pakistan border, men and boys were forced into militias that had control of camps (Terry 2002). To make matters worse, mass population movements in areas where food, water and shelter may be scarce heightens vulnerability to the rapid spread of disease, especially during the first three months of displacement, during extreme heat and cold, and in situations where the displaced population swells rapidly (Dyer 2002; Allan 2003; Thenabadu 2005). Notably, the threat of cholera, hepatitis, malaria and measles keeps aid workers on constant alert. During these outbreaks, children under the age of five often account for the highest rates of mortality (Toole 2008: 217–219).

Although Harrell-Bond (1986) and de Waal (1989) have ably demonstrated the damage that a refugee camp can wreak on the independence and self-determination of individuals (in studies on camps in Uganda and Sudan, respectively), the refugee camp can be the best way to ensure protection. Indeed, refugees are known to 'organize themselves into camp-like settings even before UNHCR and other agencies turn up' (Keen 2008: 143). Furthermore, aid agencies are often best placed to ensure that a refugee population is allowed to seek refuge in a host country, by guaranteeing that their assistance will be provided only in camp-like settings so that the population will remain in one location.

Therefore, humanitarian assistance can be a blessing and, paradoxically, a curse to refugees (Lischer 2005: 141–166). The paradox lies in the tension between needing to provide assistance to ensure the health and safety of large displaced populations, and the unintended and often negative consequences of such assistance. Assistance to refugee camps has the potential to change the social, economic and political environment, particularly when this assistance is provided by non-state humanitarian actors. Their care is essential, but it comes at the cost of further eroding the responsibility of the state to protect its own population. The next section sets out how humanitarian assistance, mainly in refugee camps, can be both a blessing and a curse by discussing two key areas in relation to the politics of health in this area of cross-border migration.

First, there is a tension between urgent medical need and the unintended ethical and political consequences. There are important questions about how much medical care should be provided by 'outsiders' in order to avoid encouraging aid dependency; this dilemma points to some of the wider implications in the relationship between politics and health. Second, the protection of vulnerable refugees who are unable to seek care from their country of origin is fraught with difficulty. While there has been a vital need for expanded strategic intervention by non-state actors in the area of humanitarian assistance – is it possible for this action to be without political consequence? Does the provision of care by a non-state actor reduce state responsibility to protect its citizens or, worse, actually assist in speeding up the expulsion of 'undesirable' populations? This highlights the central theme of this section, which is the tension between the need to address urgent needs while avoiding further harm and eroding the responsibility of states to protect their own populations.

Necessity and unintended consequences

Fiona Terry argues that when providing humanitarian assistance under conditions of instability and violence, a humanitarian actor must always consider first, whether their actions are improving the situation and second, if they are not, whether they have the capacity to act differently (Terry 2002: 206). Aid agencies, which are primarily responsible for the care of refugees in camps or camp-like conditions, have come a long way in recognizing the important role that they play in shaping the crisis they are responding to; as Toole puts it, 'the quantity of aid delivered is no longer considered a valid indicator of effectiveness; its relevance, quality, coverage, and its equitable distribution are now accepted as more pertinent' (Toole 2003: 52). Nevertheless, it is clear that significant issues remain when inadvertent politicization or deliberate exploitation is a consequence of external action to deliver urgent medical assistance to refugees.

Without doubt, the most notable example of this came in the aftermath of the 1994 Rwandan genocide, when approximately one million Tutsi and moderate Hutu were murdered by the extremist Hutu Coalition pour la Defense de la Republique (CDR), Forces Armees Rwandaises (FAR) and the *interahamwe* militia. In the wake of the genocide, which was brought to an end by the military defeat of the CDR and FAR by the mainly Tutsi Rwandan Patriotic Front (RPF), approximately two million Hutu sought asylum in Zaire (now Democratic Republic of Congo), Tanzania and Burundi (Terry 2002: 155; Stedman and Tanner 2003: 1).[1] Among the large numbers of refugees fleeing, many were civilians who genuinely believed that retribution would follow in the path of the victorious Tutsi-dominated RPF, but there were also a large number of individuals associated with the CDR, FAR and *interahamwe*. These individuals were fleeing in fear of persecution, but they were also war criminals and therefore their status as refugees was questionable.[2] In Zaire especially, and to a lesser degree in Tanzania and Burundi, large numbers of genocidal killers lived among the genuine refugee population (Adelman 2003: 96). This led to the politicization of refugee camps as they became bases for rearming and regrouping to attack the RPF. The provision of medical and other relief care to these camps, where militia were known to be diverting resources or possibly denying access to care by international NGOs, prompted questions about whether the aid agencies were doing more harm than good (Terry 2002: 2–4). This case prompted agencies and analysts to ask difficult ethical questions about the provision of scarce aid to camps where the perpetrators of violence are seeking refuge alongside civilians (Lischer 2005: 146–149; Crisp 2007: 488; Barnett and Snyder 2008: 144; Keen 2008: 126–127).

In Ethiopia, DRC, Sudan, Rwanda, Cambodia, North Korea, Uganda, Angola, Sierra Leone, Afghanistan and elsewhere the utility of medical care required re-examination in the light of the politicization of medical assistance by governments and rebels alike (Brauman 1998; Hyndman 2000; Terry 2002; Weissman 2004; Lischer 2005). The answer to this problem is that aid requires political, logistical and security support, often in the form of peacekeepers with a broad enough mandate to ensure that the camps are real safe havens. But the problem goes beyond ensuring adequate security within camps. A good example of this is Somalia in the early 1990s, where MSF was only able to operate in a surgical facility if it paid for a local security force that eventually turned on MSF after the NGO questioned the rising payments required for protection. Moreover, within the surgical facility, MSF doctors were obliged to prioritize the treatment of militia members ahead of civilians, often at gunpoint (Terry 2002: 37–38).

Experiences such as this prompted MSF France to withdraw from the Goma refugee camps in Zaire. They had mounting concerns that aid was unwittingly contributing to the strengthening of armed forces seeking refuge in the camps, who were planning to commit further mass atrocities and contribute to the continuation of conflict across the border in Rwanda. MSF France's decision to withdraw drew condemnation from other aid agencies, and indeed from many within MSF for abandoning civilians trapped within the militarized camps (Lischer 2005: 162). Fiona Terry, however, who was a member of the MSF France team in Goma, describes the dilemma of watching Tutsi children in the MSF hospital being given minimal care by Hutu staff, and MSF staff would question whether their Rwandan hospital colleagues had blood on their hands (2002: 3). The question Terry (2002) kept asking was: can a conventional medical approach that focuses on the treatment of all on the basis of need be promoted at the cost of supporting militias and even assisting continued genocide within refugee camps?

Despite this clear relationship between politics and medical aid, there remains a view prevalent among health care workers that their business is somehow removed from the political context and has few political ramifications; hence, the criticism of MSF France's actions in Goma. Reflecting the position of the ICRC, the argument is that aid can be provided in a neutral, impartial and independent space (Forsythe 2005: 6–7). ICRC's ideology of neutral humanitarianism holds that there is a clear distinction between political space and humanitarian space. For many NGOs, and individual practitioners, health care assistance should focus on assisting those in greatest need in a politically neutral fashion and such neutrality is not only desirable but possible (Anderson 1998; Noji and Burkholder 1999; Macrae 2001). From this perspective, politics is something that health care workers need to be 'aware of' but not as something that they create or contribute to (Stein 1987: 91–95; Leaning 1999a: 3, 9–11; Perrin 1999; Allotey and Zwi 2007). Even some MSF offices have been charged with regarding 'victims' and 'recipients' as helpless outsiders to the political process, a view which stems from the distinction between political space and humanitarian space (Barnett and Weiss 2008: 46–47).[3]

In the case of the Rwandan refugee camps in Zaire – when over 50,000 died from cholera within a few months – there was a huge NGO effort to assist refugees. Approximately 100 NGOs were present just in Goma at the peak of the cholera epidemic (Terry 2002: 189) and the United States deployed 3,000 troops in the same region to 'fight the ravages of cholera' (ibid. 171). This effort by humanitarian actors to restore health to at least one million Rwandan refugees (Waldman 2008: 373) had the unfortunate effect of helping to restore the capacity of Hutu militias to fight against the RPF in Rwanda. This prompted the new Rwandan government to deploy troops into Zaire, precipitating the escalation of the war. Of course, the humanitarian actors were not responsible for disarming the combatants among the refugee population or for instructing Zaire to do so, though in some of the camps some agencies – including the UNHCR – called for this, which some NGOs complained about, arguing that the UNHCR's approach made it more difficult for them to give aid (Lischer 2005: 162).

As stated earlier, the Rwandan refugee crisis was a watershed for those who had continued to believe in the unquestionable virtue of humanitarian actors and their work despite similar experiences in other conflicts such as Cambodia (Barnett and Weiss 2008: 6–7). The difference this time was the scale of the assistance and the scale of the atrocities that continued to occur. Medical assistance may have been delivered with neutral intentions but it had political consequences. The provision of aid to refugees in Goma fuelled a war economy as rebel leaders who controlled the refugee camps taxed those working for humanitarian agencies and looted humanitarian goods to sell on the black market (Terry 2002: 186–192). The refugee camps also served as 'safe' bases for the Rwandan rebels and genocidaires – and as the camps located in Zaire, Tanzania, Uganda and Burundi contributed to local destabilization, they were no longer safe for the civilians still seeking shelter there as incursions by armed groups increased (Adelman

2003). In particular, the conflict between Rwandan President Kagame (former leader of the RPF) and Hutu militias on the Zaire–Rwanda border contributed to the large-scale war between Zaire's President Mobuto and rebel leader Laurent Kabila (his son, Joseph Kabila, became President of DRC [former Zaire] after his father's assassination in 2001). This civil war expanded into a seven-state war, resulting in the highest loss of life since World War II (Roberts and Lubula Muganda 2008: 280). Over five million lost their lives, the majority civilians (Turner 2007: 3; UNHCR 2008) Therefore, what the Rwandan case demonstrates is that, while medical assistance is almost always responding to an urgent medical need and may be distributed with non-political intentions, the consequences are often political. Aid can strengthen refugee populations, particularly in camps containing combatants and non-combatants, and it can strengthen the political aims of belligerents, further wars and polarize camps.

To be sure, there are those who continue to argue that medical assistance can be politically neutral. For instance, Toole and Waldman maintain that 'solutions lie primarily in the realm of politics and economics, and are beyond the scope of public health action' for three reasons: first, health practitioners are able to document the 'magnitude of a disaster using scientifically rigorous methods'; second, once access is achieved, excess mortality can be prevented through 'implementing focused, technically effective public health programs'; and third, 'ensuring access to adequate health care should be considered a basic human right for all people', i.e. without political consequences (1993: 605). In essence, they argue that all that is needed in refugee settings is good public health; politics can stay outside the camp. Waldman (2001a) and Toole (2003) recently came back to this argument separately, with Waldman maintaining that 'providing protection while ensuring access to war-affected populations and adhering to accepted technical standards – [is] valid' (2001a: 590). Toole, on the other hand, somewhat conceded that 'the quantity of aid delivered is no longer considered a valid indicator of effectiveness: its relevance, quality, coverage, and its equitable distribution are now accepted as more pertinent' (Toole 2003: 52).

Analysis of the argument that medical assistance in refugee camps can be politically neutral and recent revisions of this argument reveal two important points. First, while medical assistance is extremely effective for conducting epidemiological surveys and delivering urgent relief in emergency situations, it is important that actors consider the political ramifications of *who* they co-operate with, to *whom* assistance is provided and *how* medical aid might protect non-combatants without also assisting combatants. Public health programmes in camps need to acknowledge and take account of the fact that political factors operate inside the camp as much as outside. Second, efforts to reduce adult and child mortality in emergency situations literally save lives but may have a ripple effect. Medical assistance may prolong conflict, medical actors may have to take sides to ensure protection of refugees within the camp, internally displaced persons (IDPs) may reveal themselves for medical assistance and then be attacked on their return home, the host country may attempt to shut down a successful refugee camp for fear of a larger refugee influx, and assistance may endanger lives if the refugee camp becomes the focus of attacks, a problem exacerbated by inadequate protection efforts by political actors such as the state, the UN or regional organizations (Lavergne and Weissman 2004; Messiant 2004; Ahoua et al. 2006).

There have been many attempts to understand these different effects of humanitarian assistance in complex emergencies in the last decade, with increasing reference to the political role that medical assistance may play (e.g. MSF 1997; Cahill 1999; Leaning et al. 1999; Weissman 2004; Keen 2008). However, there is still a tendency to assume that medical assistance is neutral and thus does not require the same critical analysis in terms of its impact on a conflict as other areas of humanitarian assistance such as the provision of shelter and food.[4] To highlight why the *politicization* of medical assistance in refugee camps needs to be better understood, I will briefly examine the recent Darfur conflict. This conflict reveals the complexity of medical assistance in refugee camps, and questions the argument that medical assistance can be considered a neutral exercise that is separate from the politics that has produced refugees in the first place.

Since 2002, Darfur province in Sudan has been embroiled in a conflict led by the separatist movements, the Sudan Liberation Movement and the Justice and Equality Movement, against the Sudanese government. The *Janjaweed* militia, which has been fighting against the separatist movements on behalf of, and sometimes with the alleged aid of, the Sudanese military, has used brutal suppression tactics against the civilians of Darfur as payback for their support of the separatist struggle. The most recent figures estimate over 300,000 dead from this conflict (Reuters AlertNet 2008), and over two million people displaced across the border of Darfur into neighbouring Chad, as well as some refugees seeking protection in camps or living rough in Kenya, Ethiopia and Egypt (OCHA 2007: 3). Humanitarian actors have confronted militarized camps, impassable border zones and chronic insecurity (de Waal 2007; OCHA 2007). Therefore, in this region, the presence of a relief worker is everything. They are vital because there is little else around to sustain life. However, the instability in Darfur has led to the border between Chad and Sudan being unsafe for aid agencies, with unprecedented attacks on relief workers (BBC 2008: 630). The insecure conditions for humanitarian workers has at times led many to question staying because assistance might be making the camps more vulnerable to attack and sometimes attacks on humanitarian workers have been perpetrated by those within the camps (Brown 2007). These dilemmas are compounded by the existence of refugee camps on the border between Chad and Darfur province that are visible and largely unprotected; people seeking refuge in these camps are vulnerable to recruitment by separatist groups, and at the same time, vulnerable to attacks by the *Janjaweed*.[5] Women and children are particularly vulnerable in this regard. While the camps offer more protection than their former place of residence, if they leave the camp for firewood or other supplies the women and children have become obvious and vulnerable targets for sexual violence by both sides of the conflict (Brown 2007). The lack of protection surrounding these camps means that these populations are chronically insecure, but the populations continue to seek the care and protection of humanitarian agencies.

The lack of a safe humanitarian space means that the relief agencies struggle to gain access to the populations in need. Providing assistance to populations that are continually on the move has required mobile health assistance units to go out and find such groups, who are often in desperate need of treatment for malnutrition. But this very act, in a situation where there is little adequate protection, increases the vulnerability of health workers and in turn, these populations, to attack. The lack of security is an obvious problem for these humanitarian actors, but so too is the fact that the majority of the medical goods and services are distributed to populations fleeing the *Janjaweed* militia, which is being supported by the Sudanese government, embroiling them in the political debate as 'taking sides' (Brown 2007: 632).[6] Once again, the key for assessing the role of medical assistance is to determine whether the assistance that agencies are providing trumps the potentially negative political impact of their presence. Darfur has revealed the excruciating uncertainties and dangers involved in assisting refugees and displaced persons without incurring unintended consequences.

Fiona Terry argues that 'pretending that the fulfillment of biological needs is a form of protection is dangerous' (2002: 52). This danger refers to the fact that, more often than not, people will flee to reach areas where aid workers are because they believe their presence will provide immediate protection. Terry argues that this perception can be dangerous because, while aid workers can treat, feed and shelter individuals, there still remain health consequences and vulnerability for those who flee to camps *en masse*, and aid agencies do not have the capacity to protect camp populations from violent attacks. In sum, people flee to camps in the belief that they will be safe havens, although those who run the camps rarely have the capacity or mandate to provide such protection. While states remain the actors most responsible for the protection of their populations and refugees, when the state has abandoned or cannot fulfil this responsibility, people turn to humanitarian actors expecting them to provide protection. This sense of protection is misplaced for three reasons. First, displaced people tend to congregate in densely populated areas, such as feeding camps or refugee camps, which allows infectious disease to spread easily among weakened and malnourished bodies (Slim 2008: 99). Second, large groups of displaced civilians make good targets for those intent on terrorizing them. The designation of 'safety zones', also known as 'humanitarian corridors', are meant to keep civilians safe from military attack while ensuring safe access to shelter, food and medical aid. However, in Sri Lanka, Rwanda, Bosnia, Angola, and presently along the border of Uganda and DRC, Chad and the Darfur region in Sudan, civilians have been subjected to attack, demonstrating that designating protection zones for civilians without adequate peacekeeping and protection mandates might place civilians at yet greater risk. The presence of humanitarian actors in this zone creates a sense of security that they simple cannot (be expected to) provide, but as chapter 5 will discuss, humanitarian agencies have always expressed concern about the politicization of aid in situations where they are dependent on peacekeeping forces for their security (e.g. Agier and Bouchet-Saulnier 2004; Crisp 2007). Third, a refugee camp with high amounts of food, medical supplies and other equipment can create a black market economy that further fuels the war economy (Kaldor 2006).

Before I conclude this section, it must be also be acknowledged that health care assistance by humanitarian agencies plays a vital role in improving the health of refugees and keeping them alive (MSF 1997; Spiegel et al. 2002; Toole 2008). In fact, the care provided in refugee camps is often better than the health care provided to surrounding local populations, particularly in camps that are in a post-emergency phase (Harrell-Bond 1986; Spiegel et. al. 2002: 1932; Singh et al. 2005). Such medical assistance can lead to refugees being (understandably) reluctant to leave the camps – even when it is safe to do so (Terry 2002).[7] Problems produced by the quality of assistance provided by humanitarian agencies have led to quite innovative developments, such as the allocation of health care to the local population to ensure that there is no resentment at the differentiation of care (Allotey and Zwi 2007), and the training of refugees as health care workers in order to build a degree of local capacity (MSF 1997: 206–222; Spiegel 2004: 713). The costs and time afforded to provide both tasks may be immense, but the benefits are significant.

One study on the Reproductive Health Literacy project amongst Sierra Leonean and Liberian women in refugee camps in Guinea found that, after attending the project, the respondents' use of modern contraception was 48% compared to 14% in the wider region and women reported discussing what they had learnt from the project with women who could not attend (McGinn and Allen 2008: 245). This may be a good indication of the positive potential of encouraging women to participate in educating other women about contraception and HIV. But these initiatives are not without their complications. Some local governments in conservative religious societies may not want local populations, especially women, to educate others about contraception. Meanwhile, a study in the DRC demonstrated that careful supervision was important to ensure the safety of patients being treated by newly trained indigenous health care workers and to avoid local staff demanding bribes on top of medical fees and the illegal sale of medications (Dijkzeul and Lynch 2006b: 72–75).

In summary, medical assistance is a vital necessity for refugees. It provides them with better health and a better chance of surviving the harsh conditions that they confront. But these services do not exist in a vacuum. The political context that has created the need for aid must then be considered in the context of health care delivery. Although the ICRC maintains that humanitarian assistance can be provided with neutrality and impartiality, it is vital to assess the political consequences that arise from delivering humanitarian assistance. Sometimes, assistance aids oppressors as well as victims and the vulnerability of citizens and humanitarian workers may actually increase to the point where a continued humanitarian presence becomes futile (Terry 2002: 53). This may not preclude the decision to provide assistance, but it is important that this and other unintended consequences are taken into account when devising health care programmes in camps for displaced persons and refugees.

Arriving in developed countries

The path of a low-income migrant or a refugee to a developed country is strewn with health (mis)perceptions that can affect their position within their new political, economic and social environment. In contrast to much previous discussion on the relationship between health and migration, I will not discuss the pull effect by which trained health care workers migrate to high-income countries, resulting in a dearth of health care practitioners in low- and middle-income countries (Diallo 2004; Nullis-Kapp 2005). Though this is an extremely important area, as evidenced by WHA Resolution 57.19 (2004) which noted with concern that 'highly trained and skilled health personnel from the developing countries continue to emigrate at an increasing rate to certain countries, which weakens health systems in the countries of origin' (WHA 2004), it has been discussed in great depth by others (e.g. Connell 2008). Instead, I will examine an area of health, politics and migration that is rather less explored. In this section, I will examine the persistent link that is made between migration and infectious disease, suggesting that this points to the underlying tensions between states' rights and individuals' rights highlighted at the beginning of this chapter. Do states have the right to deny entry to those deemed to be carriers of an infectious disease, or should health care be provided?

The speed and ease with which migrants and refugees can now travel from a low- or middle-income country to a high-income country brings with each individual's flight a closing gap in disease prevalence between these two worlds (Gushulak 2001: 261–262). Highly infectious diseases remain virulent in the regions from which most migrants and refugees emanate – Africa and Asia. These two regions have the highest prevalence of communicable diseases such as respiratory disease, TB, HIV, diarrhoeal disease, malaria and measles (WHO 2007a: 11, 18, 19). Furthermore, it is argued, travel is faster than ever before and this means that a person may not know that they are seriously ill until they have arrived at their new destination, left the airport and taken up their new residence (Rodier et al. 2000).

Carballo argues that the social, political and economic pressures that lead to people fleeing result in them carrying their ' "health" baggage with them (reflecting) those backgrounds' (2001: 272). The act of migration alone serves to increase an individual's susceptibility to disease, with human movement causing ecological change and thus emerging communicable diseases: 'refugees, displaced populations and illegal/legal workers can all bring diseases, vectors and drug resistances (e.g. anti-malarial resistance), into areas where they are not present. This may result in more severe manifestations of disease or disease at an age when the local population is immune to it' (Nathaniel 2003: 26). Cookson et al. (1998: 1) argue that 'improving the health of migrants is at the heart of reducing the public health risk to the international community from infectious disease spread by travel'. The screening of migrants and refugees for infectious diseases with the aim of preventing 'exposure', which can lead to the refusal to grant entry, has become common practice in the United States, Canada, Australia, United Kingdom and throughout Europe (Holmes and Maguire 2000: 1066; see also Fassil 2000; Palinkas et al. 2003; Vergara et al. 2003; Davidson et al. 2004; Beiser 2005).

However, evidence shows that this argument – that the unchecked flow of migrants and refugees correlates with high prevalence of particular infectious diseases in developed states – requires re-evaluation. Carballo, for example, notes that:

> [T]he immediate conclusion often tends to be that migrants bring health problems such as TB with them, the reality is more complex and is conditioned by the fact that most migrants not only come from poor health environments, but that most of them move into social situations that offer little protection against diseases of poverty. (Carballo 2001: 272)

In fact, in a separate study, Carballo notes that in the case of TB (for example) there is 'little evidence that this presents a problem for host communities, but the risk of spread within migrant communities themselves may be considerable' (Carballo et al. 1998: 937). Most migrants and refugees move straight into communities and housing where the majority of residents come from the same or similar background. Conversely, immigrants can often be in better health than their peers in the country where they are seeking permanent residency because 'good health is an advantage for getting past host countries' medical screening tests or completing hazardous journeys' (*Lancet* 2006: 1039). Therefore, the idea that migrants and refugees bring infectious diseases into the community needs further consideration.

A key aspect of infectious disease transmission across borders that has been too often overlooked in favour of the migrant link is the role of tourism and food or water exports (Rodier et al. 2000; Burnett and Peel 2001; Castelli 2004; *Lancet* 2006). There are more tourists travelling around the world (in particular from developed to developing countries) than permanent migrants, asylum seekers, refugees, returned refugees, IDPs and migrant workers added together (Gushulak 2001: 259). Each year, approximately 670 million people travel with relatively few checks to ensure that they are not carriers of disease, with at least 50 million heading from the developed world to tropical or subtropical locations for the first time (Castelli 2004: 1). A second reason why tourists pose just as much, if not more, danger to their home communities is that travellers seem to be quite uneducated about the potential health dangers in a 'different microbiological environment' (Castelli 2004: 1).[8] Risks involve failure to adhere to safe eating and drinking practices, e.g. drinking contaminated water leading to exposure to hepatitis A and typhoid fever. Lack of vaccinations, failure to practise safe sex and increasingly a failure to appreciate the risk of malaria all contribute to travellers playing a key role in spreading infectious diseases (Castelli 2004: 1). Indeed, a survey in a European international airport departure lounge revealed that 40% of the travellers could 'not correctly assess the risk of a variety of infectious disease, emphasizing the need for increased awareness in the traveling populations' (Castelli 2004: 2). We also need to consider the increased export of food and other goods from the developed world which further increases the risks (Rodier et al. 2000: 1073). For example, a *Salmonella poona* outbreak in the United States in 2008 was caused by unhygienic irrigation and packaging practices in some farms in Mexico. In another case in the early 1990s, seven people died from viral haemorrhagic fever after handling imported blood and tissue samples from African green monkeys in Uganda (Saker et al. 2007: 33).

While global infectious disease is to some extent the result of international travel, the main determinant remains poverty (Rodier et al. 2000: 1071–1073). For example, the principal sources of infectious disease lie in the disparities in immune status, the loss of income through the privatization of land leading to rapid urbanization in already poorly sanitized areas, resultant lifestyle changes, and a decline of resistance to microbes due to the inability to afford essential long-term antibiotics to tackle some highly prevalent diseases (such as TB). This is compounded by the developing world's heightened susceptibility to natural and political disasters, which provides increased opportunity for infection. Obviously, heightened travel from low- to high-income countries in an increasingly contracted time period increases the likelihood of disease spread. However, migrants and refugees are neither the sole nor perhaps the most significant transmitters.

Why, then, does the myth persist? Some argue that it persists because it is a politically convenient argument for governments to justify tight restrictions on their asylum and visa schemes (Burnett and Peel 2001; Zwi and Alvarez-Castillo 2003; Caulford and Vali 2006). Others argue that it assists in reducing the level of services that the receiving government has to provide, as the rejection of individuals on health grounds allegedly protects the 'indigenous population from an infectious hazard [more] than promoting the health of arrivals' (Fassil 2000: 59). In addition, the political expediency of rejecting refugees is more effective if 'technical' arguments such as health risks can be utilized to justify exclusion. This relates to the discussion at the end of chapter 1 where statists and globalists have increasingly securitized infectious disease, but in the case of migrant and refugee groups it could have disastrous consequences because it perpetuates existing myths about disease prevalence among these groups despite evidence to the contrary. Furthermore, such perceptions could cause those in need of treatment to retreat from seeking it for fear of authenticating host community perceptions, which then *may* contribute to the increased risk of infectious disease contagion.

For example, it has been found that the conditions that lead to refugees and migrants suffering poor health in their host country are most often *not* related to their country of origin but to the conditions they confront in their host country. While recent arrivals in Europe endure high rates of TB, studies show that as many cases occur *after* their arrival due to living in overcrowded housing with poor sanitation and difficulties in accessing health services (Carballo 2001: 272). A migrant's level of education can also be a key factor in determining whether they will seek health care (Torres-Cantero et al. 2007). In addition, medical care is often costly and time consuming, making it inaccessible to poor migrant populations (Burnett and Peel 2001, Pallikas et al. 2003; Beiser 2005) Health care schemes for migrants and refugees in high-income countries are often time specific (Carballo et al. 1998; Stanwell-Smith 2003; Vergara et al. 2003; Mjones 2005; Murray and Skull 2005). The lack of affordable and available health care is an even greater problem for those living illegally and at risk of deportation as the fear of exposing their illegal status makes it very unlikely that these populations will seek health care (Murray and Skull 2005: 27). The result is a political tension between providing unfettered health care for illegal migrants, versus the perception of being seen as soft on illegal migrants.

In summary, there is no higher correlation between refugees/migrants and the prevalence of infectious disease in developed countries, than there is with tourists returning home and the importation of goods. In fact, the health conditions for migrants and refugees can worsen on their arrival in a developed country. Despite this, there remains a common misperception that refugees and migrants spread disease, provoking responses that may create or worsen health conditions, and justifying political responses that call for more entry barriers to migrants and refugees. The securitization of migrants and refugees in linking them to the spread of infectious disease thus backfires in two distinct ways. First, it does not dissuade illegal migrants from seeking better opportunities in high-income countries, and if they become sick they will tend to delay seeking treatment due to fear of deportation. Second, as illegal migrants are willing to risk no treatment this can increase the risk of disease contagion. As Toole (2000: 126) argues, 'we must be careful that the link between mass migration and epidemics of communicable diseases is not used to impede the free movement of populations'.

Conclusion

This chapter has demonstrated how the health of migrants and refugees is shaped by political decisions made about their treatment and reception in zones of both conflict and stability, and how those decisions are informed by a tension between statist and globalist concerns. The first part of this chapter focused on the role of humanitarian assistance in shaping the experiences of refugees and displaced persons in camps. It emphasized how the work of humanitarian agencies directly impacts on the health and protection expectations of refugees. Furthermore, despite the best of intentions, the work of agencies to keep the most vulnerable people alive cannot be done in a neutral fashion and is still infused with the politics of securing the state, for example, humanitarian agencies being perceived as 'choosing sides' in a conflict. The unintended consequences, I argue, need to be better understood in the context of whether a greater number and presence of humanitarian actors create greater expectations than they can be expected to deliver. In sum, health responses to refugee crises are not neutral but become part of the political, cultural and economic context that accompanies displacement and vulnerability.

The second part of the chapter examined the reception of migrants and refugees in high-income countries. Here I demonstrated that the health status of those forced to flee their homes, or those who choose to leave, is vulnerable to political manipulation and discrimination, both of which can have a negative impact on health. The securitization of infectious disease has exacerbated a tension in high-income countries between the protection of human rights and the perceived protection of the national community from imported diseases. However, as I demonstrated, far from reducing threats by improving migrants' and refugees' health, securitized responses may actually worsen health and thereby increase the threat. Moreover, the securitization of migrants' and refugees' health status may be misplaced as these groups pose no higher statistical risk of infectious disease spread than do tourists arriving back in their home country and imported foreign food goods. This overt securitized approach to cross-border migration and disease risk leads to a neglect of alternative disease carriers and further disenfranchises already resident migrants and refugees, discouraging them from seeking health care for fear of discrimination and deportation. It also creates a false choice between protecting the state or meeting the needs of individuals.

5 ARMED CONFLICT AND HEALTH

Inter- and intra-state armed conflict, including the build-up, the duration and the aftermath, is the primary cause of long-term physical and psychological destruction for those directly and unwittingly involved. In this chapter, I will examine the relationship between armed conflict and health, focusing in particular on how politics determines the health of combatants and non-combatants during (and after) war, affecting the duration of conflicts and the prospects for peace in the aftermath. This chapter will argue that health, politics and armed conflict are deeply connected and that we need to do more to understand the role of health in determining the conduct and longevity of war. In chapter 1, I outlined the differences between the statist and globalist perspectives on health and International Relations. I highlighted how the statist perspective has the state as its primary referent, whereas the globalist generally starts with the individual. In relation to armed conflict, this tension plays out again in the question of whether the security of states or of individuals should be privileged.

As Mary Kaldor (2006) has demonstrated, most contemporary armed conflict does not conform to the old stereotype of formal state armies battling it out in a symmetrical war of attrition over national interests or territorial disputes. What Kaldor labelled 'new wars' involve a range of different types of combatant who use violence to pursue exclusionary political goals or their own economic ends. In these wars, civilian devastation is not an unintended side effect, it is a political objective and core strategy. The health of the civilian population is therefore critical to contemporary armed conflict. The purpose of this chapter is to look at how armed conflict affects health, and the responses to the challenges that it poses.

Caroline Thomas has argued that 'there may be a causal relationship between lack of material entitlement, health and education, and war' (2000: 8). Although it is difficult to prove this correlation, there can be little doubt concerning the effect of armed conflict on the health of combatants and non-combatants alike. Therefore, this chapter first analyses how we count the dead in conflicts. The death of non-combatants in conflicts is difficult to calculate at the best of times. The reporting is often based on refugee testimony, or the estimates of aid workers and military professionals. However, *who* we include in the casualty tally alters the figures greatly. Usually, those who die from famine and disease are counted as 'indirect' conflict casualties, in contrast to 'direct' casualties through direct fire. The underlying rationale of this method for counting the dead has been little analysed, yet it reveals a deeply political understanding of the deaths that are considered more important in conflict. Whose deaths are counted indicates what is most valued in determining the likelihood of a conflict's success or failure, but it also raises questions: who is protecting those dying from the indirect causes and does a humanitarian role contribute to the continuation of conflict? Answering these questions requires an understanding of what health measures are in place to protect non-combatants, who are the health care professionals in a conflict, and the role that medical care provided by combatant forces plays in the continuation of a conflict. This is the subject for the second part of the chapter. The third and final section then considers whether there is a correlation between the provision of health care and the continuation of conflict, and the importance of health care in keeping the peace in post-conflict settings.

Counting the dead

War is indelibly linked to health; it always has been. For example, the fourteenth-century siege of the Black Sea port city of Caffa ended after the Tartars catapulted in corpses infected with bubonic plague (Gould and Connell 1997: 100). The discovery of penicillin forever changed the most common cause of death for a soldier, which until that point had been infection and disease (McNeill 1998: 290; Ponteva 2001: 59). It has been estimated that since World War II there have been over 190 conflicts, and more than 90% of war casualties have been civilians (Summerfield in York 2002: 1228). Out of 191 million deaths due to conflicts in the twentieth century, half were civilians who died due to either direct (violent) or indirect (disease, malnutrition) causes (Sidel and Levy 2003: 516). Thomas Weiss (2007: 69) argues that in this century 'civilians have continued to represent an increasing percentage' of those killed in conflict. Mary Kaldor

argues that 'new wars' are characterized by the tendency of warring
factions:

> to avoid battle and to direct most violence against civilians . . . At the begin-
> ning of the twentieth century, 85–90% of casualties in war were military.
> In World War II, approximately half of all war deaths were civilian. By the
> late 1990s, the proportions of a hundred years ago have been almost exactly
> reversed, so that nowadays approximately 80% all casualties in wars are
> civilian (Kaldor 2006: 107)

The fact that more civilians than soldiers die as a result of war brings to
the fore the question of how we should count war's casualties. This is
important because numbers shape policy priorities.

The question of who to count revolves around whether deaths due to
malnutrition, forced removal and loss of means of sustenance, and the
withdrawal of medical facilities due to the conflict, should be counted
alongside battle-related deaths (Collins 1993; Gustafson et al. 2001). These
deaths are brought about by the conditions caused by war, but are 'indirect'
because they were not caused by violence itself (Garfield and Neugut 1997;
Small Arms Survey 2005). On top of this, the causes of indirect death are
more complicated as they are partially determined by economic and health
conditions *before* the conflict, and not exclusively by the conflict itself
(Iqbal 2006). Particularly in the case of disease, even if it is linked to
deprivations caused by the conflict, is it difficult to know whether this link
is causal or just a correlation (Garfield and Neugut 1997; Terry 2000). We
know that direct civilian deaths due to violence can prolong conflict, as
people may be encouraged to engage in retribution, or the conflict may
end due to the incapacity of one side to keep fighting. But what of indirect
deaths? How do they create conditions for conflict to continue or end?
We know very little about this, and it could be argued that this is largely
due to the primary focus being on conflict at the 'state level' rather than
examining the correlation between conflict and health at the 'individual'
level.

The Small Arms Survey (2005) reveals that the relationship between
direct and indirect deaths can be complicated by location of the conflict.
In the 2003 Iraq war and 1999 Kosovo conflict, the direct death rate was
85% and 100%, respectively. In contrast, between 2000 and 2004, conflicts
in sub-Saharan Africa had a direct death rate of only 23.6% (Small Arms
Survey 2005: 253–254). One important point from these figures is that the
conditions in a state *before* the conflict greatly affect the impact that a war
will have on the civilian population (Iqbal 2006). In Kosovo, for example,
the majority of the sick population suffered from 'developed world' diseases such as heart disease and diabetes. Infant mortality and maternal

mortality rates were not comparable to those seen in the developing world and therefore the primary health concern during the conflict was providing food aid to a generally healthy population, deprived of the essentials over a relatively short period due to the war (Small Arms Survey 2005).

If we use direct death measures only, our understanding of the impact of conflict diminishes. As we noted earlier, the people dying from indirect causes in sub-Saharan Africa vastly outnumber those dying from direct causes in Iraq and Kosovo (Small Arms Survey 2005). However, we need to be careful not to conflate proportional death rates with absolute numbers. Even across Africa, the story differs from conflict to conflict. Darfur receives a higher per capita amount of humanitarian assistance than the DRC (IRC 2006). This could be attributed to the direct death tally: in 2003, the proportion of direct deaths in Darfur was between 11.6% and 29.6% while in the DRC it was 2.7–16.5%, but the DRC lost approximately 200,000 people due to direct causes compared to Darfur's 70,000 (Small Arms Survey 2005: 236–237, 245–246). Two other points make the picture still more complex. First, due to inconsistent mortality reporting systems, the death rate may be underestimated and this is an even greater problem when trying to count indirect deaths during a conflict (Small Arms Survey 2005: 238–239). Second, as mentioned above, the proportion of direct/ indirect deaths does not give us an accurate picture of the overall devastation that conflict causes. The DRC has lost approximately 5.4 million people from the recent six-year conflict, 75% of whom were children, women and the elderly who died from preventable diseases and malnutrition (Coghlan et al. 2008). Even though these deaths were not due to acts of fighting, the war's presence was a strong contributing factor. The societal consequences can only be measured once the fighting stops, but one thing we do know is that in the DRC the children who survive the war will have become familiar with death and destruction at a very personal level in their young lives (Coghlan et al. 2008). How this trauma will impact on future attempts at conflict resolution and peace-building is yet to be discovered.

Distinguishing between direct and indirect deaths can, however, play an important role in helping to craft strategies aimed at preventing, or mitigating, the health effects of conflict. The proportion of direct and indirect deaths can be used to determine where the humanitarian response should be directed (Iqbal 2006). It has even been argued that 'standardized mortality and morbidity surveillance systems should be established to provide the basis for all early [humanitarian] interventions' (Cobey et al. 1997: 314). The number of indirect deaths can also be predicted sooner if actors record the level of health care that was available to 'vulnerable' populations before the war (Small Arms Survey 2005: 255; Toole et al.

2006: 452). To assist in building evidence of the causal relationship between war and indirect deaths, Banatvala and Zwi (2000), the Small Arms Survey (2005: 238–241) and Woodruff (2006) all argue that a partial solution is to create surveillance mechanisms that provide more detailed mortality data as opposed to the simple calculus of 'direct' and 'indirect' deaths. Such a mechanism would categorize the causes of death more clearly, allowing for links between pre-conflict and conflict phases to be established, thus illuminating whether it was the conflict or the conditions before the conflict that most impacted on a particular population. Of course, such detailed surveillance is usually not possible in conflict zones, which is why such interventions have not occurred or are piecemeal (agencies count deaths where it is relatively safe to do so, see Small Arms Survey 2005: 236–237; Coghlan et al. 2006). Building mortality surveys that could chart the cause of non-combatant deaths more precisely would better inform the humanitarian response by directing agencies to areas in greatest need and direct political attention to the conflicts that require immediate safe corridors for humanitarian access. In the long term, such data may allow us to start building a better picture of the devastating impact that health has on the trajectory of conflict.

For now, though, it is important to note that increasingly civilian deaths outnumber combatant deaths in conflict and that civilians die in many different ways that are difficult to identify and trace with precision. Deaths of civilians have continued to outnumber deaths of soldiers since World War II (Holdstock 2001: 184). This is in spite of advances in the Geneva Convention, specifically the Third Convention and Second Optional Protocol, which recognize the duty of protection of non-combatants in international and intra-state conflict, respectively. It is also in spite of unprecedented levels of humanitarian assistance in and surrounding conflict settings (Tong 2004). Acknowledging the difference between indirect and direct deaths is important because continued and widespread civilian deaths can shock the conscience of international society and build evidence of violations of the Geneva Conventions (Bellamy 2006). Seeking to understand how conflicts operate and continue at the 'individual' rather than 'state' level may allow new modes of enquiry that feed into broader themes such as the war economy and the politics of new wars. Furthermore, greater efforts to trace indiscriminate attacks on civilians by armed groups can, in turn, lead to demands for international engagement to find political solutions to end such conflicts (Bellamy 2006). However, with the partial exception of the intervention in Somalia in 1992, slow unyielding deaths due to starvation, disease and lack of access to health care have tended not to attract the level of attention needed to provoke international intervention.

The role of humanitarian agencies

It is no coincidence that during the same period in which there has been a dramatic increase in indirect civilian deaths during armed conflict, there has also been a dramatic increase in the number of humanitarian agencies working in conflict zones. The collapse of the state, particularly in civil conflicts, has resulted in an incapacity or unwillingness of states to provide essential care to their populations during conflicts. This has led to humanitarian agencies filling the caretaker void that has been abandoned by the state. Without doubt, the presence of humanitarian agencies has prevented the indirect death toll in conflicts such as DRC, Angola, Somalia and Afghanistan from being even higher. However, humanitarian agencies do not save lives in armed conflicts in a political vacuum. As discussed in chapter 4 in relation to refugee camps, the consequences of filling the caretaker void – traditionally the responsibility of the state – means that these agencies are contributing, willingly or not, to the political conflict. The existence of medical facilities in a particular conflict zone, treatment of particular populations, hiring of local staff and distribution of aid all contribute to the economy and continuation of war (Terry 2002). Keeping in mind Mary Kaldor's (2006) argument – that civilian devastation is not an unintended side effect but a political objective and core strategy vital for modern conflicts – it is important to evaluate how the work of humanitarian agencies contributes to the political dynamic in such conflicts.

The proliferation of humanitarian agencies in situations of protracted civil war has contributed to three key developments involving health care delivery. First, the development of the Sphere Project (in 1997–98) provided technical guidelines and a Humanitarian Charter that set out minimum standards for NGOs in refugee and conflict crises. Concerns with Sphere, raised by MSF in particular, have been focused on whether technical measures have been overly emphasized and have overshadowed the need for greater commitment to political efforts to end crises. Second, the relationship between military and humanitarian actors has become particularly contentious since the 'war on terror', and specifically the increase of US Department of Defense activities in this area since November 2001. This debate dovetails with broader ethical concerns such as, when military forces become involved in aid, does aid then become a legitimate target in war? Finally, the combination of these two concerns has led to a split in the academic field about the precise role that humanitarian actors play in conflicts. There is a 'narrow line [for public health professionals], particularly in direct participation activities [in war zone], between protecting and serving people, and enabling the war effort to move forward' (Levy and Sidel 1997: 389). With the increased militarization of aid and, at the same time, an increased emphasis on technical targets for measuring the effectiveness of aid (rather than political efforts for ending the war), the last part of this section will discuss whether humanitarian actors are still able to claim that the good they achieve outweighs the potential negative consequences of their presence. This discussion dovetails closely with the relationship between necessity and unintended consequences discussed in chapter 4. The proliferation of actors responding to conflict-induced health crises also reflects the complications that arise from the tension between the roles and duties of state and non-state actors in the system of 'global health governance' as discussed in chapter 2.

Sphere

The Sphere Project was developed after the humanitarian disaster that befell Rwandan refugees in Goma following the 1994 Rwandan genocide (see chapter 4). It was found that a lack of consistent minimum standards for NGOs contributed to a failure to recognize the risk of cholera outbreaks in the camps, along with problems of peace and security within the camps (Riddell 2007: 329; Keen 2008: 144). The Sphere Project produced a handbook of *Minimum Standards in Disaster Response* – technical measures for increasing the effectiveness of humanitarian aid, including areas such as minimum daily nutrient intake, the size of tents and access to water (Riddell 2007: 329). The handbook also contained a Humanitarian Charter and Code of Conduct, to which humanitarian agencies were to adhere. The Humanitarian Charter and Minimum Standards were to become a measure of accountability by which NGOs' effectiveness would be measured. The Humanitarian Ombudsman Project, now the Humanitarian Accountability Project International (HAPI), was then set up under Sphere to publicize grievances with NGOs (Tong 2004: 181). While some see this as a measure of ensuring accountable NGO activity in conflict and refugee zones where exploitation and inefficiency could go unnoticed (Riddell 2007: 341), others argue that Sphere has important flaws (e.g. Terry 2002; Tong 2004; Keen 2008).

First, Jacqui Tong argues that her agency, MSF, chose not to participate after the first phase of Sphere's development (1997–1998),[1] because the project's emphasis on technical approaches to crises neglected 'the fact that in most crises, the majority of death and suffering during conflict and/ or displacement is caused by the lack of political will for ensuring the welfare and protection of a vulnerable population' (2002: 177). She argued that those who share closer relationships with donor governments or have specific communitarian beliefs (e.g. religion) will have less trouble adhering to Sphere, which is increasingly being adopted by donor governments as a measure by which to determine whether NGOs should or should not receive funding (Tong 2004: 178, 183). However, if a humanitarian agency considers impartiality and independence to be its most important assets in the delivery of aid, particularly in conflict settings, close relationships with donors – and donor support based on adherence to technical standards alone – will cause additional problems. Moreover, Sphere leaves NGOs vulnerable to donor demands and, in turn, the politicization of aid (Terry 2000; Tong 2004).

Furthermore, the danger with technical standards is that they are minimalist and do not allow for adaptation, which means that strict adherence to Sphere could make conditions worse in some conflict settings. Fiona Terry argues that the problem with Sphere is that, more often than not, meeting technical requirements is not the critical issue; instead the problem comes from agencies competing with each other and undermining each other's work. In conflict settings, this may create the 'space' for warlords to monopolize camps and expand their war economy as they siphon off surplus humanitarian supplies and sell them on the black market, demand taxes or fees from agencies for renting warehouse space, and create inequality among refugee, IDP and local groupings (Terry 2002: 13–16). MSF has argued that their problem is not with technical standards for humanitarian work but 'the problems rested with linking quality and accountability to technical standards. This can be exemplified by the hackneyed example – "there are a sufficient number of wells but women are raped to collect water"' (Tong 2004: 182).

Overall, the concerns about Sphere revolve around the extent to which we think that humanitarian agencies influence the conduct and continuation of conflicts. If, as Riddell (2007) and Waldman (2001b) argue, the Sphere guidelines are just about how many litres of water each individual should have access to per day, then there is little to quibble about. However, if Terry (2000), Tong (2004) and Keen (2008) are right, and Sphere starts to bring in – little by little – conditionalities that NGOs must abide by, then NGOs are no longer working according to assessments of what each situation requires but what the guidelines and donors say. Moreover, if an agency cannot meet the standards or if the situation makes it impossible to meet the standards (e.g. after the earthquake in Pakistan in 2006), should they just withdraw or pick and choose the standards that they can meet (Keen 2008: 145)? How does this improve accountability and transparency – the overall purpose of Sphere? As for HAPI allowing grievances to be reported, as Terry argues (2000: 21), it is highly unlikely that an individual in a refugee camp or trapped in the middle of a war zone would report an NGO even if they knew about the reporting procedure. What impact has Sphere had on the humanitarian actors present in conflict settings? Ironically, given its opposition, MSF more than meets all the Sphere technical guidelines, as do UN agencies and other large NGOs such as Oxfam and Save the Children (Riddell 2007: 341). What remains unclear, and this is the core concern of Sphere's critics, is whether NGOs follow Sphere because these guidelines represent the best response to the situation they are working in, or because this is what their donors expect. The greater danger is that Sphere may deter NGOs from providing care beyond minimal expectations and may encourage governments to think that technical standards for humanitarian assistance represent a useful substitute for political measures to tackle the underlying causes of the conflict and human distress (Terry 2000, 2002; Tong 2004). International political action to end a conflict remains often more important for saving lives than tents or oral rehydration therapy.

Moreover, concerns about donor interference in the activities of humanitarian agencies are not without merit. Aid may be conditional on commercial opportunities that constrain the actions and independence of humanitarian agencies (Riddell 2007: 100). If a major donor to a particular NGO is an enemy of the state that the NGO is working in, then the workers and their actions may not be seen as neutral or impartial by local actors (Lavergne and Weissman 2004: 155). The idea of the neutral humanitarian actor, i.e. an actor that has no interests and no impact on the political context or conflict, is a myth (Terry 2002). Actors will always be trapped in subjective and deeply political understandings of who is vulnerable, who needs saving, who is at fault and who needs to be kept away from camps and medical clinics. The concern is, as we will see below, when donors start to interfere with the actions of humanitarian agencies, as Sphere has the potential to do, that humanitarian space is put at risk and this can risk lives in conflict settings.

Militarizing aid

After 9/11 (the terrorist attacks of 11 September 2001), the United States and its allies intervened in Afghanistan in November 2001 and Iraq in March 2003, and often referred to humanitarian assistance and reconstruction as part of its strategy for winning the 'war on terror' (Weiss 2007: 146–147). For example, US Secretary of State, Colin Powell, described NGOs working in Iraq as 'force multipliers' (Weiss 2007: 146). Likewise, UK Prime Minister, Tony Blair, called for a 'military-humanitarian coalition' in Iraq (Shetty 2007: 377). The US Department of Defense has also sought to link humanitarianism and combat operations, stating that humanitarian actions can assist combat operations due to both having the long-term goal of fostering 'democratic institutions and a robust civil society' (Bristol 2006: 384).

Some NGOs, such as Oxfam, MSF and ICRC, have expressed concerns that such activities are 'blurring the lines between what the military is supposed to do and what the humanitarian community does . . . If the military were doing an adequate job providing security, their basic competence, there would be no need for them to be filling in gaps in humanitarian/development coverage resulting from insecurity' (James Bishop, InterAction's Director of Humanitarian Policy and Practice, in Bristol 2006: 385). But what is wrong with the military providing assistance to communities where there is too much instability for humanitarian workers to operate safely? The problem is 'operational effectiveness', argues Nathaniel Raymond of Oxfam America (Bristol 2006: 385). When warring factions are unable to distinguish between civilian humanitarian workers and the military, they do not worry about making the distinction and simply target both. This makes aid work increasingly dangerous and it is no surprise that the number of aid workers killed has increased over the past few years as they have been accused of aligning with the United States (Bristol 2006: 385). As the ICRC argues, 'actions presented as humanitarian are [all] becoming suspect, perceived – rightly or wrongly – as part of a wider strategy to defeat an opponent or enemy' (Bristol 2006: 386). Or, as Weiss (2007: 147) points out, the 'manipulation of humanitarian values to facilitate militarism' is illegitimate and as we have seen in recent years it is costing aid workers their lives.

The problem here is that the distinction between impartial humanitarian work and politicized rebuilding work is being blurred. Blair's and Powell's comments 'serve only to increase the perception that all western NGOs are merely extensions of foreign policy' (MSF UK Director, Jean-Michel Piedagnel, in Shetty 2007: 377). Indeed, MSF attributes its decision to withdraw from Afghanistan in 2004 after the murder of five health workers to its 'perceived links with US forces' (Shetty 2007: 377). Likewise, Oxfam's Iraq policy adviser, Jo Nickolls, argues that the militarization of aid 'denies the possibility of neutrality by simply vanishing it away' (Shetty 2007: 377).

Meanwhile, what is to be made of the aid agencies who are only too happy to blur the line between military and humanitarian agendas, as has been alleged against CARE America in Afghanistan and Iraq, who argue that they support the political goals of rebuilding (Shetty 2007: 377)? There are two potential concerns here. The first is that humanitarian efforts are constrained when NGOs closely align themselves with military and political forces for protection. Military and political objectives are rarely the same as humanitarian objectives. While it is one thing for humanitarian work to create unintended political or military consequences, it is another practice altogether to side with a military or political actor to deliver aid. Second, when humanitarian actors embed their aid delivery projects within military operations, they undermine the claims of neutrality, impartiality and independence made by all humanitarian agencies working in that particular conflict because it becomes harder for non combatants and enemy forces to identify which agencies are not 'force multipliers'. However, in response to these concerns, the US government has argued that the correlation between alleged links to Western governments and attacks on NGOs is overstated. The Director of Civil-Military Medical Affairs in the US Department of Defense (Health Affairs) argues that 'it's a very unsafe world for these organizations to be operating in. I think a lot of them come under attack whether they're affiliated with a military or not' (Daniel Tarantino in Bristol 2006: 385).

The other dilemma in militarizing aid is the role of military medics – military personnel conducting humanitarian actions in conflict settings. In these situations the crux of the question, similar to that facing humanitarian agencies, is whether medicine can ever be delivered in a conflict zone in a neutral manner. Sidel ostensibly argues that this can be the case (1997: 287), while Gross argues that 'any military role, combatant or noncombatant, inevitably violates the principle of nonmaleficence when the military operations of which medical personnel are an integral part harm others. Medical personnel are not in any way neutral or above the fray' (2006: 293). However, Sidel posits that the combatant role of medical personnel is not the same as that of soldiers, for under the Geneva Convention they and their facilities are to be immune from attack.

A case that highlights the tension of military medical units playing humanitarian roles is that of the Australian medical contingent deployed to Rwanda in 1995 to provide health care as part of the United Nations peacekeeping force, UNAMIR. In the aftermath of the Rwandan genocide, the victorious RPF had surrounded an IDP camp at Kibeho. In April 1995, Australian medical personnel witnessed increased tension within the camp and the presence of two RPF battalions surrounding the camp. Occasional shots were fired into the camp by the RPF and food deliveries were blocked over a five-day period. On 22 April, with an approaching thunderstorm, IDPs ran for shelter and the RPF, mistaking this action as an attack, fired into the crowd – killing 130 people (Friedman et al. 2003: 344). The Australian medical team worked on the injured until, a few hours later, the RPF opened fire again. All UN staff sought cover during the night, and the next morning Australia medical personnel counted 4,000 dead IDPs and treated 650 wounded (Friedman et al. 2003: 344). In this instance, military medics played an important role as witnesses to a massacre and in providing medical care to the victims. The extent to which their presence limited the extent of the massacre is unclear, but one of the primary concerns for the Australian Force Medical Officer (FMO) in the immediate aftermath was to *prevent* his troops seeking revenge on the RPF for the bloodshed. The FMO recognized that one of the tensions in the deployment of military medics in humanitarian zones was that they had the capacity not only to treat, but also to injure, and that maintaining a distinction between the two required careful vigilance. In other words, the neutrality of military medics will always be in tension with their other identity as combatants who have the wherewithal to take sides.

Another concern with proactive military medical engagement among civilian populations is that it further exacerbates the vulnerability of that community through association, and blurs the distinction between medicine and military strategy. An African proverb best illustrates this tension: 'when two elephants fight, it is the grass between them that suffers most' (Slim 2003: 494). As noted above, even in humanitarian missions the choices confronting military medics in war can be (inevitably) different to the choices confronting humanitarian agencies (Slim 2003). Indeed, for a military medic, the concept of neutrality may be at odds with the reason for being in the conflict in the first place. This, in turn, explains why some humanitarian actors argue that the military should never assist in the provision of humanitarian assistance – because humanitarian actions conducted by the military will inevitably have political objectives (Gross 2006: 206–209), whether it be promoting stability by lending credibility to the government in power, undermining the government by promoting the intervention, or the use of force to protect one group rather than another.

The underlying dilemma of militarized aid is that co-operation with the military may enhance aid agencies' capacity to deliver health care in the most difficult environments and ensure some protection for civilians seeking such assistance. However, enhanced capacity bought through co-operation with the military comes at the price of perceived neutrality. The concern of NGOs such as Oxfam and MSF is that, when the neutrality of one agency is questioned in a conflict, so too are the other agencies working in the conflict. This impacts on agencies' ability to travel in a conflict zone to reach IDPs and other civilians in need. The protective label of humanitarian actor is removed once an NGO is perceived to be 'taking sides', and this not only endangers the lives of aid workers but also civilians who seek treatment from these agencies. This is why the same NGOs argue that military medics should not extend beyond treating and assisting their own wounded.

Minimizing harm

Knowing when the provision of relief is contributing to harm minimization and when it is no longer doing so can be difficult for humanitarian agencies to determine. Relief agencies can have a 'dark side' (Slim 1997: 256). While they are always there because of the violence of others, this does not mean that everything they do is necessarily beneficial. It all depends, Slim (1997: 251) argues, on how the agency sees its responsibility to act in the given situation. One agency may see its actions as good in themselves and that the 'goodness' of that action is not dependent on the consequences that follow from it (*deontologists*). On the other hand, another agency may argue that the consequence of the action is all that matters for it has wider impact (*consequentialists*). Slim's (1997: 251) categorization of the humanitarian role in conflict as being either deontological or consequential best sums up the debate about the role of the humanitarian in conflict.[2] The deontologist, in the context of providing health care in a war zone, would argue that it does not matter who is being treated because everyone is human and the treatment is given in good faith. However, a consequentialist would maintain that who is being treated is vital for understanding the consequences on the prolonging of war (Slim 1997: 251). So how do humanitarian actors navigate their way through a moral calling to alleviate the suffering of fellow human beings, but avoid inadvertently prolonging suffering?

For humanitarians, one thing is certain: 'the age of innocence, if there ever was one, is over' (Weiss and Hoffman 2005: 297). The role of testimony is one area that especially highlights the tensions that a humanitarian worker faces in the field. For example, what is the duty of an NGO to give testimony to the International Criminal Court (ICC) if a witness to genocide and mass atrocities? MSF was threatened in west Darfur by a local militia who told them that if the UN provided a peacekeeping mission 'we would be considered part of that western front, and a jihad would begin' (Shetty 2007: 377). NGOs are increasingly placed in the middle of conflicts, particularly due to the increased number of IDPs who remain in conflict zones and require humanitarian assistance (Cohen 2007). As a result, direct reporting of conflicts and of the actions being taken by both sides leads agencies such as MSF, ICRC, Save the Children, Oxfam and other UN humanitarian offices to become important testimonial actors. But how does this role fit with the need for humanitarian workers to be impartial and neutral in conflicts so as to ensure access and safety? The ICRC has resolved this dilemma for them by stating that it will not provide evidence to the ICC. The ICRC places strict limits on its engagement with political or legal institutions, arguing that its role in reporting atrocities and human rights abuses to ensure the upholding of international humanitarian law must be balanced against the need for access to future conflicts without placing their workers in danger (Forsythe 2005: 273–278).

Access may require that an agency *not* take a political position. But how does this fit with the agency's broader mandate to protect civilians from harm? Neither position is perfect. On the one hand, humanitarian actors that faithfully report what they see may make warring factions more conscious of the need to adhere to international humanitarian law in order to avoid an Interpol arrest warrant to appear at The Hague. On the other hand, warring factions may either assume that all humanitarian actors will report their actions and therefore they strike at anyone who witnesses them committing an atrocity, or refuse all humanitarian access to civilian populations. Either way, it demonstrates the tension between seeking to immediately prevent harm against considerations of the long-term consequences of a particular action.

To make matters more complex, the role of humanitarian aid in conflict settings treads a fine line between prolonging the war through the provision of assistance to the war effort (Leaning 1999b: 81–93; Messiant 2004: 124; Weiss and Hoffman 2005: 302–304), and saving many innocent people from suffering (Toole et al. 2006; Djikzuel and Lynch 2006b). More often than not, humanitarian assistance is not enough to stem the violence (Terry 2004; Lavergne and Weissman 2004; Coghlan et al. 2006). This is where the argument between the consequentialists and deontologists picks up again.

Hugo Slim (1997) argues that, in such contexts, humanitarian actors should critically assess whether they are making a positive contribution. In particular, he argues that there are two questions every organization must ask itself: first, 'is the organization secure in the belief that its actions are always good in themselves?' and second, 'does the NGO believe it needs to have a sure grasp of the wider consequences of its programmes to be certain of the goodness of its work?' (1997: 251). However, it is difficult for agencies to answer these questions by themselves (Weiss and Hoffman 2005: 205–206). Humanitarian agencies need intelligence (hard data) – 'substantial information-gathering and comparative analyses on the range of incentives and disincentives that are attractive to non-state actors [and some states – depending on who is the source of the conflict]' (Weiss and Hoffman 2005: 307).

This brings us back to the question of how we assess civilian casualties of war, as discussed in the first section of this chapter. Humanitarian workers need to know who needs assistance and who will benefit most from the assistance that they can provide. Weiss and Hoffman concede that if they cannot get this information to form an accurate picture of who they are helping or need to help, or, if their assessment shows they will do more harm than good, NGOs may have to withdraw and effectively abandon those whom they could have helped. We saw this reality played out as described by Fiona Terry in relation to Goma in chapter 4, and similar arguments have been made about aid to North Korea (Terry 2004), Sudan (Lavergne and Weissman 2004) and Africa in general (de Waal 1997). As such, aid agencies need to adopt strategies to deal with this tension and this requires them to realize their political role in conflicts. Aid agencies can no longer deny that their presence is political (Duffield 2001), though this can lead to reprisals against staff, as Slim (1997) and MSF (Shetty 2006) point out. Nor can agencies deny the need sometimes to confront the impact that their aid is having on the conflict (Weiss and Hoffman 2005: 310). They may also need to consider engaging warlords and the state to ensure the delivery of aid – but this is fraught with dilemmas and pitfalls (Weiss and Hoffman 2005: 311).

Overall, the tension for humanitarian workers in understanding whether they are prolonging a conflict or keeping innocents alive is best dealt with by confronting the tension between consequences (consequentialists) and good deeds 'in the present' (deontologists) (Keen 2008: 145–146). Delivering aid to those who need it can 'become a radical political act that challenges power structures and exploitation. In particular, confronting – rather than disguising or ignoring – the blocking of relief leads donors and NGOs towards an analysis of the political forces that may be trying to produce a disaster' (Keen 2008: 145–146). Most crucial for navigating this dilemma is that a humanitarian agency should not provide aid as a bargaining chip, or for any reason other than to save lives: 'by definition, any aid given to induce political, religious or economic compliance is not humanitarian aid: the only compliance that should be sought for humanitarian aid is with conditions that will ensure that aid is given to those most in need' (Terry 2004: 106). Commentators and practitioners need to better evaluate humanitarian aid – including medical assistance – to ensure that it is humanitarian in focus and not a thinly veiled attempt to advance a political agenda, or an inadvertent contribution to the political agenda of one side in the conflict. This is difficult when humanitarian actors are sometimes the only ones standing between the life and death of civilians, but as Lavergne and Weissman argue: '[H]umanitarian actors are heavily implicated in the abuse of humanitarian action. It is their duty to ensure that their actions conform to the principles they claim to uphold' (2004: 161). Therefore, we need to better understand how states can be persuaded to fulfil their duty to protect their own populations in these situations, how to reduce the situations where civilian deaths outnumber those of combatants, and how to relieve humanitarian agencies of being the sole actors seeking the protection of civilians.

In summary, the proliferation of actors seeking to provide health care as part of a broader humanitarian effort has arisen in part because the number of civilians in conflict who face the risk of death due to disease, famine and isolation has grown. It is important to recognize the political character of humanitarian activities – whether overtly political as in the case of humanitarian agencies embedded in military units, or covert, where agencies are unwittingly contributing to war economies and contexts. While causation is difficult to prove, there is clearly a connection between the proliferation of 'new wars' (Kaldor 2006), the prolonged suffering of civilians in conflict zones and the proliferation of humanitarian actors. The age of innocence is over and humanitarian agencies must assess their role in saving lives and ending wars with a keener sensitivity to the political repercussions of their actions. However, the ultimate responsibility is on those engaged in the violence to seek political solutions at the peace table.

The war is over . . . if you can survive it

What role does health play in ending war and keeping the peace? Until recently, while health provision was treated as part of the reconstruction effort, it was not considered to be an activity that could actually have the same positive impact as the rule of law and security sector reform in securing the peace (Jones et al. 2006). However, with increased awareness of how humanitarian aid can change the direction of war (see above), analysis of the post-conflict setting has come to indicate that health plays an important part in winning the peace.

This section will first discuss the relationship between good health and sustainable peace-building. We need to understand how and why the availability of health care for civilian populations is linked to increased stability in post-conflict settings. Then, the section will go on to highlight two complications that follow with health care provision in a post-conflict setting. First, success is dependent on the level of health care that existed before the war began (Iqbal 2006; Jones et al. 2006). Second, the provision of health care during and after war is dependent on ascertaining how many health professionals remain in the country (Deely 2005; Wakabi 2007b), and then how to make the transition from health care as provided by aid agencies (often during the conflict) to a self-sustaining indigenous system (post-conflict) (Poletti 2004; Dijkzeul and Lynch 2006b).

Restoring health in a post-conflict environment

Good health is vital for rebuilding a state (Deely 2005: 138). But how important is health for the establishment of peace and who needs to be providing good health? A recent RAND study evaluating a number of post-conflict reconstruction efforts since World War II found that health is not given sufficient credit for the success of reconstruction efforts (Jones et al. 2006). This study showed that there is a significant correlation between health and security (Jones et al. 2006: xvii). If there is an improvement in life expectancy, birth and death rates, infant mortality rate, infectious disease rates and malnutrition, then post-conflict operations are significantly more likely to succeed (Jones et al. 2006: xviii–xix).

The principal reason why health contributes to the restoration of peace is because it is a 'superordinate goal' that 'transcends the separate goals of parties to a conflict, and that can best be achieved when the parties join efforts' (Santa Barbara and MacQueen 2004: 384). When a ceasefire is negotiated for a day in order to vaccinate children against measles or polio, both sides agree to it because these 'days of tranquility' or 'corridors of peace' (Grant 1997: 17–18) create a benefit that transcends the separate goals of the warring parties. This is particularly the case when the act is led by a perceived 'neutral' actor such as ICRC or UNICEF.

The RAND study shows that the correlation between nation-building and health is positive when assistance is co-ordinated and includes support for infrastructure (Jones et al. 2006: 278–279). Health, RAND maintains, is an independent variable that can win the 'hearts and minds' of the local populations, and efforts to build health provision should always be seen as the work of the government rather than outside actors (Jones et al. 2006: 281). On the other hand, failure to improve health – either due to inability to reach medical staff or lack of improvement to basic conditions (such as clean water, access to shelter and food) – can demonstrate an overall failure to create a secure post-conflict environment and increase the political vulnerability of the ruling government. For instance, in Iraq, insecurity often made it impossible for health care staff or patients to get to their local clinic, and a lack of military personnel to guard water pipelines as they were repaired resulted in slow improvements to health and increased anger at coalition forces. The RAND study suggests that 'lead agencies' and 'mission coordination' can provide solutions for these situations where there is not enough security to continue the health restoration projects (Jones et al. 2006: 287). The study argues that problems in Iraq, Afghanistan and Somalia related to poor co-ordination between peacekeepers, NGOs and international organizations such as WHO (Jones et al. 2006: 288–289). Another study has demonstrated how tension between local staff and international staff in a post-conflict setting can create difficulties in assigning health care responsibilities (Deely 2005: 131). Of course, some of these agencies argue that the central problem was not a lack of co-ordination, but the broader politicization of aid by donor governments which impaired the independence that these same agencies relied on (Shetty 2007).

Therefore, access to health care is not only important for creating the perception of post-conflict stability, but it actually assists with the creation of a stable and functioning post-conflict environment. The RAND study demonstrates an important link between the provision of health care and success in post-conflict nation-building. The provision of health care contributes to political stability and security, establishes a positive state presence across its territory, and lays the foundations for economic recovery. Thus, complications connected to the provision of health care in a post-conflict environment can affect the overall success or failure of post-conflict reconstruction. I will now highlight two possible complications.

Health before and after the war

Indirect deaths during conflict (deaths due to preventable illnesses, failure to vaccinate young children against diseases that can be fatal, and malnutrition) are often attributed to the level of adequate health care available before the war (Ponteva 2001; Iqbal 2006; Jones et al. 2006). However, a note of caution must be attached to these arguments: although the provision of health care before a conflict is significant, conflict itself has a massive effect on a country – regardless of the level of health care available pre-war.

A recent and prescient example of the impact of the pre-war system and the effects of war on it is provided by Bosnia-Herzegovina. Before the conflict, which began in 1992, Bosnia-Herzegovina enjoyed universal and centralized health care. After the fall of communism, this universal health care system remained intact. The newborn mortality rate was 14.5 per 1,000 (in Western Europe it was 9.5) and there was a relatively good number of medical staff as a proportion of the population (Konttinen 2001: 233; Horton 2003: ch. 4; Simunovic 2007). In the aftermath of the war,

Bosnia's health care staff relative to population had declined by 40% (Konttinen 2001: 235), infant mortality rates went up to 24.7 per 1,000, and there was a rapid increase in drug-resistant tuberculosis (double the rate pre-war) and hepatitis A (Horton 2003: 134). In addition, thousands were wounded by landmines or sustained other war injuries (Kotinnen 2001: 236–237) and the country was plagued by the health consequences of the mass rape of women, which included illicit life-endangering abortions, sexually transmitted diseases and suicide (Arcel 1998). The only upside to all of this, argues Horton (2003), is that because of the level of surgical training among those doctors who remained in the former Yugoslavia some important discoveries were made in trauma care – particularly in the reconstruction of limbs after war injuries (Horton 2003: 135).[3] Obviously, such surgical care is less possible in war zones that lack Bosnia's medical infrastructure, such as Afghanistan, Somalia and southern Sudan (Leaning 1999b: 85–86; Lavergne and Weissman 2004: 149–150; Wakabi 2007b). Nonetheless, it is important to note that Bosnia's relatively sophisticated health system did not insulate it from the health costs of war.

Of course, where health systems are not so strong the number of indirect deaths (in particular) will be significantly higher. For example, in the DRC 5.4 million people are now estimated to have lost their lives during the six-year conflict. Only 10% of these deaths were due to direct violence (Coghlan et al. 2008: 1). The remaining deaths have been due to starvation and disease. Even before the conflict, the DRC had a poor health care system with high child and maternal mortality (Turner 2007; UNHCR 2008). The DRC's national crude mortality rate (CMR) of 2.2–2.9 deaths per 1,000 per month is 57% higher than the average rate for sub-Saharan Africa (Coghlan et al. 2008: iii). There has been a persistent increase in the DRC's crude mortality rate since the war began in 1998, with children accounting for 47% of deaths even though they only make up 19% of the total population (Coghlan et al. 2008: iii). Therefore, such sharp differences between these figures and the Bosnian experience can be attributed in part to their very different pre-conflict health capacities.

The relationship between violent conflicts and health is indisputable and closely linked to the level of human security that existed pre-war within the given community (Iqbal 2006: 634). Good health relies on the financial capacity to seek it, the social right to have it, a safe environment to go to the clinic, and work to pay for medical services (People's Health Movement et al. 2005: 257). Often, pre-war environments are characterized by prolonged diversion of economic resources from public health to military use, which impacts negatively on health so that by the time of conflict early signs of deprivation may already be starting to appear in child mortality figures and maternal deaths, as happened in the DRC (Sidel and Levy 2001: 211–214).

Palmer and Zwi (1998: 237–239) go so far as to argue that the status of women in society is also a critical pre-conflict factor. With large numbers of girls and young women dying from malnutrition, reproductive and maternal complications and communicable diseases, as occurred in Somalia, southern Sudan and Afghanistan (to name a few), as well as their education being compromised due to not being allowed to attend school, the 'crucial role women play in maintaining the structure and function of families and society diminishes' (Palmer and Zwi 1998: 239). The potential for women to serve as peaceful negotiators, health care workers and distributors of food and shelter in refugee camps has been well documented (e.g. MSF 1997; Nakaya 2004; Ashford 2008), but it is vital to further explore whether women's pre-conflict status affects the health of the nation and is a likely contributor to prolonged conflict.

Another unexplored area is the impact of higher deaths within a particular demographic on the peace-building process. Spiegel and Salama (2000) found that in Kosovo there was evidence of a higher than usual risk of mortality for Kosovar Albanian men aged over 50, largely due to their traditional role as head of household and guardian over family lands. Their higher than usual mortality was on the one hand due to deliberate targeting by Serbian forces – in that removing the traditional 'head' of the Kosovar Albanian family weakened the family unit – and on the other, the inability or refusal of elderly men to leave family land which meant that they were often victims of shelling and, after the war, family members' inability or lack of desire to return left these men uncared for (Spiegel and Salama 2000: 2208). We still know very little about the effects of direct targeting of particular populations – such as killing senior Kosovar Albanian men, the mass rape of women in Bosnia and DRC, and the very high death toll of children in the DRC – on peace-building processes.

From an International Relations perspective, such knowledge is essential for determining the early warning indicators of conflict and the essential post-conflict factors that are more likely to sustain peace. The provision of health care before a conflict can be an important indicator for determining the path of difficulty in reconstructing health care after conflict. For instance, we know that there will be a higher indirect death toll in conflict settings where health care was already minimal. Therefore, a key complicating factor in a post-conflict reconstruction effort is the quality of the health care service *before* the conflict began – this is a good argument for proposing that health care should be adopted as an early warning indicator for systems that predict conflict and mass atrocities. From a peace-building perspective, it would also indicate whether the task is going to be focused on restoring security so that existing staff and supplies can resume, such as was the case in Bosnia and Iraq, or whether, as in the case of the DRC and Afghanistan, the task involves building infrastructure from scratch. In addition, the quality of health care before a conflict is also important for indicating which demographic may require immediate health care in the post-conflict environment. We know that particular demographics may be more vulnerable during the conflict and their vulnerability can prolong a conflict. Although it remains understudied, securing the health of a particular demographic may be important for restoring security to local communities if these individuals are the primary source for food, security and money in the family unit. Understanding the nature of a health care system before a conflict, and the role that the state needs to adopt afterwards, is crucial for securing the health of individuals. It may also determine the trajectory and likelihood of sustainable peace.

Health as a public good

Usually, public health is already straining under the weight of budgetary pressure and individual affordability before the outbreak of war. While crucial for the short-term survival of individuals, the immediate rush of international aid agencies to respond to urgent humanitarian needs after the outbreak of war can have long-term effects on the rebuilding process. For instance, in recent years, some donors and other development advocates have increasingly argued against the provision of free health care in conflict settings (Poletti 2004: 19). The World Bank and International Monetary Fund in particular argue that health care needs to be an 'auto-finance system' (Dijkzeul and Lynch 2006b: 4) in conflict and post-conflict settings. Cost recovery for 'publicly financed goods' such as health should continue on the basis of 'user pays' (ibid. 8). While clearly a product of the Bank's free market agenda (see chapter 2), the rationale for this is twofold. First, the population will have difficulty in transitioning from a (free) health care system (provided by aid agencies) to a user-pays health care system, thus it is best to minimize the upheaval in the delicate period of post-conflict rebuilding by instituting user-pays from the outset. Second, in order to ensure that local health care workers stay in the country, there needs to be wage continuity during the conflict. As warring states are rarely able to pay health care workers, it is best that health care is provided through a market economy system to ensure the flow of income and thereby reduce the migration of health care workers.

In conflict, however, cost recovery becomes difficult due to rapid economic decline, the oppression of particular populations, and 'patronage politics' (Dijkzeul and Lynch 2006b: 9). While these problems mitigate the use of user-pays in conflict settings, the World Bank still argues that the user fees system is better for the post-conflict reconstruction effort. The benefits of user-pays are that it increases the sustainability of health systems and the likelihood of local health workers remaining as they see a viable future income for themselves if they stay; user-pays reduces the tension between those accessing aid and those unable to, and enables local training and capacity-building (ibid. 2–4).

Obviously, this concept of user-pays is controversial. How, for instance, are orphaned children, the elderly and women without the means to earn an income to pay for health care during conflict (Djeddah 1996)? What happens when even under this system local health care workers do not earn enough to support their family (Ferrinho et al. 2004)? What does this user-pays system say about the principle of humanitarianism (providing assistance to those who are most vulnerable and unable to access it) (Keen 2008)? Finally, does a user-pays system actually assist post-conflict recovery (Dijkzeul and Lynch 2006b: 9)? I will briefly consider some of these points in more detail.

One study on local health care in eastern DRC showed that the effects of 'user-pays' depends on the manner in which it is implemented (Dijkzeul and Lynch 2006b). The same study criticized UNICEF and MSF for providing free health care, arguing that it does nothing to build a sustainable health care system (ibid. 9). However, if the purpose is simply to maintain local health systems and nothing more than that – what Dijkzeul and Lynch refer to as the 'hands-off contract' approach (2006b: 3) – then aid delivery *is* preferable to user-pays. Despite their criticism of UNICEF and MSF, Dijkzeul and Lynch (2006b) acknowledged that user-pays has yet to recognize the vital difference between emergency relief and capacity-building. Furthermore, user-pays lacks the essential humanitarian ingredient which ensures that access to health care is available to all (particularly those most at risk of disease – the poor and IDPs), and that proper procedures are adhered to (regarding treatment, use of medications, etc.) (Poletti 2004).

In a recent study, Dijkzeul and Lynch compared four different approaches to local health capacity-building projects in the eastern DRC run by the International Rescue Committee (IRC), Medical Emergency Relief International, Merlin, and Association Regionale d'Approvisionnement en Medicaments Essentiels (ASARAMES). They found that of the four agencies, using four different capacity-building projects, none used the 'hands off approach' and 'to differing degrees, they all carry out capacity building and supervisory control. They all rely on cost sharing and the provision of free drugs and other medical supplies. The organizations have improved access with lowered fees and, in two cases, coupons for the indigent [poor]' (Dijkzeul and Lynch 2006b: 3). Furthermore, none of the local staff was found to favour providing health care for free: 'they argued that it could lead to abuse of the health system, take away patients' dignity and would not be sustainable in the long run (especially not when the international organizations leave)' (Dijkzeul and Lynch 2006b: 59).

The study concluded that 'in a chronic crisis, in some circumstances no user fee should be implemented in order to remove financial barriers (for example, during epidemics or larger population displacements) or there should be a reimbursement system' such as the use of vouchers (Dijkzeul and Lynch 2006b: 68). Security and economic conditions, donor requirements and the quality of local counterparts all had a significant impact on the degree to which the four agencies could rely on the intense supervision and capacity-building approach. However, Dijkzeul and Lynch (2006b: 68–70) were able to identify nine important insights about how the four agencies dealt with these issues:

1   Access increases when fees are lowered for children aged 5–15.
2   If NGOs reimburse clinics that treat impoverished patients, the number of impoverished patients treated by the clinic is sustained (no dramatic increase in patients above what the clinic can cope with).
3   When reimbursement for an impoverished health system is provided, cost recovery amounts to only 30–45% of the health facility's overall operational costs. External support is therefore essential to continue treating the impoverished; but the overall income is from user-pays.
4   External support from an NGO is essential in chronic crises to ensure continued access.
5   Donor support will continue to be necessary in the near future (in eastern DRC).
6   Balancing the needs of donor and local health management will be successful if both parties agree to reduce user fees, but still support the practice of user fee system.
7   The size and location of the health zone affected the security of the staff and those being treated. The larger the area that the clinic had to look after, the more difficult it was to ensure security for staff and that patients could reach the clinic safely.
8   Fees must be adapted to the economic and security situation of the population. Fees needs to be advertised so that the patient is aware of the user-pay system and to ensure that health care providers do not attempt to charge more.
9   It is hard to identify who *isn't* using the service and, therefore, what total number of the population is and is not accessing the service (making it difficult to plan for post-conflict reconstruction).

There are at least three problems with the user-pays system, even in this case where alternatives were provided for those unable to pay. First, there was no clear definition by any of the four agencies as to what 'impoverished', or needy, meant and this meant that there were different user-pay fee schedules across the agencies (Dijkzuel and Lynch 2006b: 36–66). From a reconstruction point of view, this meant that different groups will benefit more or less from different agencies. This lack of coherence impacts the effectiveness of user-pays. Differing policies on who can be defined as needy, which determines who should pay for their health care, creates problems for the redevelopment of a national health system.

This leads to the second problem, which is that there is no hard evidence that user-pays actually assists in the post-conflict restoration of health services and it may potentially do more harm (Poletti 2004: 22). For example, post-conflict Burundi is still heavily reliant on donors such as IMF and the World Bank. At present, if patients are unable to settle their bills, hospitals have been known to detain patients. Moreover, the public health system is vulnerable to corrupt practices and many go without essential medical care (Wakabi 2007a: 1847). In response to this problem, the Burundi government decided to remove the user-pay system from certain medical services, mainly birth delivery and children's health services. This led to a 75% reduction in maternal deaths and 50% reduction in neonatal deaths (Wakabi 2007a: 1847). The government eliminated user fees for maternal and pediatric health care with the assistance of WHO, UNICEF, the UN Population Fund and World Food Programme. However, since the implementation of this programme, Human Rights Watch has alleged that Burundi has been 'punished' by the World Bank and IMF with a reduction in its health care budget from $15 million in 2006 to $11 million in 2007 (Wakabi 2007a: 1847–1848).

Obviously, differentiated mandates among international organizations leads to tension and contradiction in assisting states with their health care policies – as discussed in chapter 2. However, in a country struggling to prevent the recurrence of civil war – where the majority of the population lives on less than $1 a day, 1,000 per 100,000 women die in childbirth and there is an infant mortality rate of 114 per 1,000 births – the call to re-evaluate how user-pays enhances the chances of progress for this post-conflict state is not without merit, especially given the evidence that the situation in Burundi improved after abandoning user-pays. If we go back to the situation in DRC, the vast majority of deaths in this conflict were caused by preventable and treatable illnesses, with the mortality rate at its highest in the eastern provinces where Dijkzuel and Lynch (2006b) conducted their study (Coghlan et al. 2006: 44). The utility of a user-pay system must be measured against the capacity for it to enhance the survival rates of those living in such dire circumstances. Evidence to date suggests that it does not.

The third problem with user-pays is the emphasis on local health workers. There is a long record of trained health professionals leaving conflict zones (Toole et al. 2006: 458–500). It is clearly important to stem this tide. Programmes to do so need income to be viable, and this can be immensely difficult to organize as government spending on health typically declines during conflict, especially civil war, a problem compounded by the fact that portions of territory may be held by rebels and most populations cannot afford to pay the taxes necessary to rebuild the public health service. To make matters worse, retaining local medical staff as the main providers of medical care during the conflict increases their risk of harm. Harm can manifest in two distinct ways. First, health care providers in general are increasingly becoming victims of conflict (Deely 2005: 127; Shetty 2007). If humanitarian agencies are subject to accusations of siding with one group or another, mistaken for armed convoys, or targeted in case they provide crucial testimony to the international community about mass atrocities, it is obvious that local health workers will face similar threats. Therefore, the idea that the tide of health care worker migration can be stemmed through user-pays needs to be balanced against the reality that health care workers may also leave due to fear for their personal safety. For example, during the Mozambique conflict between 1980 and 1992, health workers were 'systematically targeted, kidnapped and killed by RENAMO fighters' (Deely 2005: 126). In southern Sudan in 2001, a pro-Khartoum militia – the South Sudan United Movement (SSUM) – entered a MSF hospital treating forty soldiers and demanded that all be removed from the hospital. All of the soldiers hospitalized were considered by the MSF to have been forcibly recruited – the youngest was twelve years old. MSF negotiated with SSUM for a MSF doctor to accompany the SSUM to decide case-by-case whether each patient was fit to leave (Lavergne and Weissman 2004: 149). Twenty-four were taken away (five had already fled during the night), including one who had to be carried out on a stretcher. However, MSF staff also risked their own lives to protect the local hospital staff from being attacked for treating 'enemy' soldiers, who were threatened with being forcibly recruited into renewed military service (Lavergne and Weissman 2004: 150).

In a strict user-pays system, there may be much less international presence at a hospital like the one above in Sudan, significantly increasing the risks to local staff and encouraging their flight. Also, it should be mentioned that a user-pays system does not prevent local health care workers from being agents of harm. Local health care workers may take sides, give preferential treatment and exploit supplies for their own gain and survival (Toole et al. 2006).

Ultimately we need to ascertain what sort of assistance can best build health capacity for the future. The user-pays approach is presented as necessary for ensuring that post-conflict health care is sustainable long after the donors have left and the agencies have moved on. However, the system does not resolve the three problems already noted. First, there appears to be no criterion or guide on who should be exempt from user-pays, in the sense that 'impoverished' would apply to many in the aftermath of a war. The problem of residual tension when some have to pay but not others does not appear to have been considered either, yet this could be quite an important factor depending on the demographic make-up of the region in a post-conflict setting. Second, it is hard to build health care capacity based on the income from user-pays in countries such as the DRC, Sierra Leone and Burundi, where the majority of the population are impoverished and have little income to contribute in the form of taxes or health care fees. Third, it is not clear that user-pays achieves what it sets out to do. There is little connection between health indicators, the retention of health care workers, and whether or not a user-pays system is in place.

In sum, there is an important correlation between access to health care and nation-building. The provision of health care indicates progress, security and stability and gives the state a positive presence. All this serves to increase the population's faith and support in the post-conflict rebuilding phase. Yet there remain two important complications that can affect progress in health care rebuilding. First, the level of health care available before the conflict has a large role in determining the health care infrastructure challenges after the conflict. Second, health policy and financial investment from global actors may emphasize responses that may further divide already fragile populations into those who can afford health care and those who cannot, such as user-pays systems. From a capacity-building perspective, if health care infrastructure is already weak, then a system such as user-pays will be ineffective for improving capacity. Large foreign investments are still the key for health care infrastructure development in post-conflict settings, but consideration must be given to the local factors that determined the level of health care available to all populations before, during and after the conflict, if sustainable peace is the aim.

Conclusion

This chapter has highlighted the relationship between health, politics and armed conflict. As in other chapters, the tensions between statist and globalist perspectives is all too evident, this time in relation to who should be protected, whose death should be counted in the conflict tally, and who should be served by the long-term aim of peace. This chapter assessed how we count the dead in war and noted that deciding who to count as a victim of war has political consequences: counting the dead more accurately allows a better understanding of the costs of war and the challenge of building peace. However, the complex relationship between conflict and health has been starkly revealed by an increase in the number of actors that now engage in humanitarian action in conflict zones and the dilemmas that they confront. The rise of 'new wars' (Kaldor 2006) and the dramatic increase in civilian deaths as a proportion of the total indicates that states continue to abandon their duty to protect their populations from harm. This situation has given rise to humanitarian actors seeking to provide the protection that the state cannot or will not provide. However, humanitarian actors cannot protect individuals without political consequences. From resistance to the idea of 'minimum standards' for disaster response as specified in the Sphere guidelines to the increased militarization of aid in the post 9/11 environment, many humanitarian actors see their 'space' being encroached on by politics. Increased calls for humanitarian actors to 'embed' their work into military operations are being resisted by many, but not all, in the sector. As a result, the perception of humanitarian actors as neutral actors – fundamental to the establishment of humanitarian space – is under threat (if, indeed, it was ever safe). This means that agencies are having to choose between, on the one hand, the risk of staying and endangering the lives of aid workers and some civilians, and, on the other hand, the risk of leaving and abandoning those who are most vulnerable. The end of innocence is the realization that humanitarians do not need to be carrying a gun to have an effect – for good or ill – on conflict escalation.

Finally, health care is also linked to the success of ending war and keeping the peace thereafter. Keeping local health care staff in the country and encouraging a user-pays system (as opposed to reliance on humanitarian actors for medical aid and care) is a core part of the World Bank and IMF efforts to build sustainable health care systems. However, this approach is deeply flawed. The flight of local health workers is not just a product of inadequate wages. The implementation of user-pays may not always be effective in providing health care, and poor health in a post-conflict environment can be related to the lack of poor health care *before* the conflict. Income from user-pays cannot resolve these entrenched health infrastructure gaps, and there is much at stake in post-conflict environments if health infrastructure gaps continue without remedy.

There is much yet to be explored in understanding the relationship between health, politics and conflict but what is clear is that the relationship is embedded with political actors, perspectives and objectives that can explain why conflicts start, how they continue, who survives and who gets to rebuild the peace. We need to do more to address the problem of how global actors can satisfy the needs of vulnerable civilians within conflict zones without inadvertently relieving states of their responsibility to protect their populations from harm.

6 INFECTIOUS DISEASE

The health issues that are prioritized by domestic and international policy makers impacts on the choices available to those suffering from poor health and lacking adequate health care. The health choices available to AIDS victims, refugees, women and those caught in conflict are determined by the level and type of health care provided to them. Moreover, the ability of the world's marginalized to fight for political and economic freedom is correlated, at least in part, with the political priority that has been accorded to their health. The identity of *who* gets to prioritize particular health conditions and health care programmes has undergone massive change in recent years, associated with globalization and the emergence of global health governance. Economic and capacity inequalities between states mean that certain actors – such as donor states and philanthropic agencies – heavily influence the health priorities of aid recipients (see chapter 2). Of course, donor states are to a certain degree self-interested actors, and therefore the policy priorities they promote may reflect their interests at least as much as those of the recipient states. Meanwhile, the growth of private and non-state actors has increased the number of actors that influence health policy and engage in health care delivery, making the overall picture more complex. As I noted in chapter 1, the area where both these trends are most noticeable is the effort to prevent the spread of infectious diseases across state borders. While renewed interest in this subject might provide evidence of the emergence of globalist concerns – prioritizing the needs of the individual according to a human security ethos – the manner in which it has been pursued, via the language and logic of 'securitization', demonstrates the continuing power of statism. Financial resources and political attention has been focused primarily on diseases that are considered likely to cause illness on a global scale (and including the world's wealthy states), such as influenza, rather than diseases that are highly infectious but limited to particular geographic and economic demographics, such as scabies.[1] This chapter evaluates how global concern with the spread of infectious disease has become a matter of 'high politics' and explores the consequences.

First, though, it is important to clarify the terms used in this chapter. Communicable diseases are diseases that are passed from one human to another (via human to human contact, insects, animals or the environment). All communicable diseases are infectious, but not all infectious diseases are communicable.[2] Infectious diseases are caused by a micro-organism and thus some micro-organisms may cause high mortality or disability (such as a flu virus), but sometimes will only infect one or two persons (as in the case of anthrax or smallpox bacteria). Diseases that are both communicable and infectious may be spread by an insect vector (e.g. malaria and dengue fever, both spread by mosquitoes) or by an animal host (e.g. rabies, spread by a viral zoonosis that resides in domestic and wild animal species including dogs, foxes, mongooses, raccoons, skunks and bats). Humans can be infected and infect each other in a number of ways. In the case of rabies, transmission may be through saliva from an animal's mucous membrane or from a bite that transfers the virus to the human's open cut. Cholera, on the other hand, is a disease spread by a bacterium (*Vibrio cholerae*) which spreads through the ingestion of food or water that is contaminated with faeces. When there is poor sanitation, crowded living conditions and unprotected water sources, cholera (and malaria, measles, and dengue fever) can reach epidemic proportions very quickly, as occurred in Zimbabwe in 2008–9. Securitization language mostly focuses on infectious diseases, rather than the broader category of communicable diseases, largely because the diseases that preoccupy Western states with their security concerns are either highly contagious or linked to biowarfare.

At least 4,500 children die every day from communicable diseases that are preventable[3] (WHO 2007b: 4). In 2001, access to uncontaminated food and clean drinking water could have prevented the deaths of two million people due to infectious diseases (Kindhauser 2003: 6). In 2001, AIDS, tuberculosis and malaria accounted for 33% of deaths due to infectious disease, i.e. 5.6 million people, and in the same year another 5.8 million died from diarrhoeal disease and respiratory infections (Kindhauser 2003: 6). These five diseases accounted for 78% of the total infectious disease burden in 2001 and little had changed by 2007 (UN 2007). Indeed, between 2002 and 2007, forty new infectious disease strains emerged and there were some 1,100 reported epidemics of infectious disease, the outbreaks occurring primarily in low-income countries or those enduring complex emergencies (Grein et al. 2000: 97; WHO 2007b: x). The average annual number of dengue fever cases has doubled in the last forty years, in part due to the reduction of vector-borne disease control programmes over the same period (WHO 2007b: 18). A multidrug-resistant strain of tuberculosis is now also on the rise due in part to failure to alleviate poor living conditions in the geographic regions that are most vulnerable, and in part because the disease spreads easily among HIV-infected patients (Farmer 2005). An additional concern is that WHO's statistics cover only about half of the world. WHO collects cause of death statistics from all of its 192 member countries, yet in 2007 WHO had only 56% (sixty four countries) of the data for 2004 and 2005 (WHO 2007a: 14). This means that for 'more than a fourth of the world's population – largely located in Africa, South-East Asia and the Middle East', there is no data to indicate the disease burden accurately (*Economist* 2006: 14; WHO 2007a: 14).

As I noted in chapter 1, the global spread of infectious disease is increasingly evoked as a security threat (Bower and Chalk 2003; Fidler and Gostin 2008; Price-Smith 2009). In particular, there has been increased reference to the threat that an infectious disease pandemic such as influenza or an epidemic such as AIDS may pose to national security (de Waal 2006: 79–83; Gostin 2008: 89–90). These diseases are equated with economic destruction and political instability, and even depicted as a threat to healthy populations in the developed world (Peterson 2006). However, while the securitization attempt has meant that particular infectious diseases have reached the realm of high politics, a great number of communicable diseases – particularly those that are most likely to remain in poor, low-income countries – are not receiving the same level of attention despite the fact that some of these diseases contribute to a greater number of deaths per year. This is a direct product of the fact that securitization helps create political priorities sometimes, as in this case, at the expense of other equally pressing concerns that are not securitized. The cause of inertia in relation to the broader category of communicable disease is largely down to the fact that some of these diseases, such as rabies and cholera, are hardly likely ever to reach epidemic proportions in countries that have relatively sophisticated health care systems. Nor do such diseases call for treatment programmes that entail 'extraordinary' measures traditionally associated with the 'high politics' solutions. Such diseases require long-term measures related to the alleviation of poverty. Therefore, they remain neglected by high politics.

This chapter will map how concerns about emerging and re-emerging infectious diseases (REIDs) have come to inform the securitization of infectious disease. In particular, the appearance of REIDs among communities in North America and Western Europe has increased the level of attention given by those states to the 'threat' that certain infectious diseases may pose.[4] As awareness of infectious disease has increased among

Western governments over the past two decades, responses have largely centred around three questions. First, do infectious disease containment measures require global co-operation, as opposed to the traditional emphasis on state-led public health measures? Second, if the former is required, will the securitization of infectious disease succeed in persuading states to co-operate in order to address the problem? Third, will securitization further erode policy interest in the totality of the global disease burden (Heymann 2003: 117–118; Anon. 2004b: 1640)? This chapter will address each of these questions by tracing how political responses to the perceived threat of infectious disease outbreaks, particularly among Western states, resulted in revision of the International Health Regulations (IHR), a legal framework that is meant to strengthen collective action to prevent and contain the spread of infectious disease. The chapter will conclude by questioning whether the IHR represent a new attempt to synthesize the health needs of both individual and states, or whether they effectively securitize infectious disease at the expense of other health needs (especially the broader category of communicable disease).

Infectious disease as a security threat

The association of infectious disease with state security is not new. As David Fidler and Mark Harrison argue, since the first International Sanitary Conference in 1851, states have long perceived infectious disease as a threat to their population, to their ability to trade and to accept migrant labour (Fidler 2003b; Harrison 2004: 103). In fact, Andrew Price-Smith argues that we must go back even further to regard the 'effects of infectious disease on structures of governance', which he demonstrates by examining a number of specific pathogens and their 'deleterious economic, social, and political effects on politics, from ancient times [e.g. typhus during the Peloponnesian War, plague and destruction of Byzantine Roman empire] to the early twentieth century' (2009: 35–36).

However, it was the 1851 Conference that, according to Fidler, spawned the term 'microbialpolitik' (1999). Microbialpolitik is the combination of two forces:

> forces compelling States to co-operation on infectious disease control and to develop international law on this problem, and those forces that restrict the outcomes of such co-operation and the scope of the resulting international law. The forces that propelled States to co-operate were fear of new diseases and economic losses caused by other States' reactions to infectious diseases. (Fidler 1999: 52)

Fidler charts how scientific developments along with economic self-interest and balance of power politics led to the international sanitary conferences in the late 1800s and early 1900s waxing and waning in the interests of the (mostly) imperial states that attended the conferences. The real movement came when infectious diseases started to have a large impact on military forces, and new technology in travel meant that individuals could travel faster by steamship and railway, causing diseases to spread faster (Fidler 1999: 55–56) However, before the introduction of the 1951 WHO's International Sanitary Regulations (ISR) (renamed in 1969 as International Health Regulations; IHR), the power of international sanitary conferences had been relatively minimal in terms of impact on state behaviour (McNeill 1998: ch. 6; Fidler 1999: 58).

The IHR were introduced in 1969 in order 'to ensure the maximum security against the international spread of diseases with a minimum interference with world traffic' (Fidler 1999: 61). Only a decade later there was some confidence among public health officials that the risk of infectious disease had been reduced. It was widely believed that new treatments, vaccines and knowledge of microbes would lead to the eradication of infectious disease as a major cause of death by the end of the twentieth century (WHO 2000a: 1). This optimism proved to be short-lived. The outbreak and rapid spread in the 1980s of HIV/AIDS, followed by the resurgence of stronger microbe-resistant pathogens causing malaria, TB, meningitis and dengue fever, was compounded by the fear that bioterrorists might use deadly pathogens as a weapon to inflict mass casualties (Sanders and Chopra 2003: 106). New infectious pathogens (emerging infectious diseases; EIDs) have been discovered at the rate of one per year over the last two decades (Merianos and Peiris 2005: 1250).[5] In the last ten years, serious infectious disease discoveries have included Ebola, Lassa and Marburg haemorrhagic fevers in Africa, variants of Creutzfeldt-Jakob disease in Western Europe, meningococcal meningitis W135, Nipah virus in Malaysia and the West Nile virus in North America (Heymann 2003: 106–108).

Then in 2003 there was an outbreak of a new respiratory disease, severe acute respiratory syndrome (SARS), and in the same year, human cases (though animal-to-human, not human-to-human) of H5N1 avian influenza. These events led some to claim that the world will not be able to escape a pandemic influenza outbreak in the next few years that could kill anywhere between 2 and 12 million people (WHO 2006). All of these developments served to increase calls for particular infectious diseases, including AIDS, influenza, weaponized smallpox and anthrax, and to a lesser extent drug-resistant tuberculosis, to be identified as a threat to national security (WHO 2000a; Brower and Chalk 2003; Fidler 2004a; Gostin 2004; WHO 2007b).

Such arguments have not gone unnoticed by Western governments (Aginam 2005b). During the 1990s, awareness of the threat that particular infectious disease outbreaks could pose to citizens' health, as well as to economic and political stability, encouraged Western governments in particular to develop responses in national security terms. Acute awareness that Western states were not immune to this threat was raised by outbreaks such as the West Nile virus and drug-resistant infectious diseases such as TB, measles and meningitis in the United States and United Kingdom, as well as the outbreak of SARS in Canada. In the rest of this section I will briefly demonstrate how the United States, Australia, Canada and Europe's invocation of particular infectious diseases as a security threat increased by the turn of the century and how each of these states have increasingly seen containment at the source as the best response. The result, of course, has been the prioritization of certain infectious diseases over others in the realm of 'high politics', with the result that the diseases that continue to cause high mortality and morbidity remain neglected and are found among the poorest and disenfranchised.

The United States has been a keen participant in disease surveillance and response since the mid-1990s (Fidler et al. 1997). While the US Department of Defense (DoD) has had overseas laboratories investigating infectious disease outbreaks since the 1960s, the Global Emerging Infectious Surveillance and Response System (DoD-GEIS) was established in 1998 with renewed capacity and reach (Fearnley 2008: 70). The DoD-GEIS overseas infectious disease research laboratories were given the capacity to be located in over twenty countries at any given time (Chrétien et al. 2006: 538). The mobile laboratories were set up for 'responding to outbreaks of epidemic, endemic and emergent diseases' (Chrétien et al. 2006: 538). Their location in the DoD, as opposed to within USAID or the Centers for Disease Control demonstrates how seriously the US government considered infectious disease preparedness and response as a key element of its national security strategy. Further evidence of American urgency in containing infectious disease outbreaks was demonstrated by its political and financial support for the WHO's infectious disease surveillance notification network – the Global Outbreak Alert Response Network (GOARN) and Strategic Health Operations Centre (SHOC) located at WHO headquarters to monitor and report on infectious disease outbreaks (Burns 2006: 769).

Financial support for monitoring systems such as SHOC and containment mechanisms such as the DoD mobile laboratories indicates that the United States has taken the threat of infectious disease seriously (Fidler

2004b; Enemark 2006; Fearnley 2008: 69–76). David Fidler suggests that there are three reasons for the United States' increasingly securitized response to infectious disease. The first is the threat of bioterrorism (Fidler 2004b; Fearnley 2008: 70). Even before the anthrax attacks in the United States in late 2001, the US government had been warned of the threat posed by deliberately released pathogens into cities via subways, movie theatres or dispersed by turbine engines, water or sewerage ducts (Brower and Chalk 2003: 10–12). In 1996, President Clinton identified the need to bolster US biodefence capabilities, as evidenced by investment in the DoD-GEIS mentioned above (Chrétien et al. 2006: 538; Enemark 2006: 55–56). The United States also increased its financial contributions to multilateral infectious disease surveillance operations. For example, the United States committed to the G7 + Mexico Global Health Security Initiative in 2001, where signatories agreed to 'strengthen global surveillance and outbreak response' to prepare for biological terrorist attacks (Kindhauser 2003: 17).

Second, Fidler argues that the US government started to connect the evolution of naturally occurring infectious diseases with globalization, coming to the view that such interconnectedness between poor and wealthy travellers increased the risk of infection spreading across the globe (Fidler 2004b; also see chapter 4). Within the United States, public health systems were encountering infectious diseases that they had either previously thought eradicated, or had not seen before. The West Nile encephalitis, new strains of measles, multidrug-resistant tuberculosis, malaria and cyclosporiasis have been diagnosed in the United States, arriving through imported water and food goods or arriving with citizens returning from overseas travel (Smolinski et al. 2003: 1). In a report for the US Institute of Medicine, it was argued that the United States needed to enhance the 'global capacity for response to infectious disease threats, focusing in particular on threats in the developing world' and take a 'leadership role in . . . a system of surveillance for global infectious disease' (ibid. 8–9).

Finally, Fidler (2004b) suggests that the development of US government interest in infectious disease was related to the realization that infectious disease epidemics in foreign countries could threaten US national interests. For example, the United States played a key role in introducing the UN Security Council resolution that linked HIV/AIDS to future state failure and regional instability in the developing world because of the high risk it could pose to soldiers and skilled citizens. Earlier, a 1998 paper entitled *Reducing the Threat of Infectious Diseases* announced that the 'capacity of all nations to recognize, prevent, and respond to the threat of emerging and re-emerging infectious diseases is the critical foundation for an effective global response' (USAID 1998: 1). Waiting for the outbreak to arrive and then responding should be the last resort, argued USAID. The first line of defence is 'prevention, treatment and control programs' before the disease reached US shores (USAID 1998: 2). USAID recommended that containment was the best defence and that this could be done through developing a strong infectious disease surveillance capacity. The crucial factor, argued USAID, was improved co-ordination between international health organizations and that states be willing to report high outbreaks of infectious diseases (USAID 1998: 3–5).

Among policy makers in Australia, Canada and the European Union, McInnes and Lee have noted a similar realization of the perceived need to plan for infectious disease outbreaks, whether naturally occurring or caused by bioterrorism (McInnes and Lee 2006). The emerging consensus has been that such an outbreak would constitute a threat to national security and thus support for global health security has become a stronger feature in the national policy of these states (McInnes and Lee 2006: 7).[6]

In Australia, particularly since the outbreak of SARS and H5N1's deadly re-emergence in 2003, defence strategists, academics, economists and politicians have all warned of the potentially serious consequences if the government does not prepare at the federal level for a pandemic (Lee and McKibbin 2003; White 2005; Hartcher and Garnaut 2006; Richardson 2006). For example, the Australian Treasury has stated that a potential outbreak could cause a 'recession about half the size of the Great Depression' (Hartcher and Garnaut 2006). Both the Australian Attorney-General's Department and the Department of Industry, Tourism and Resources websites have links to 'Being Prepared for an Influenza Pandemic', stating the steps that individuals, companies and hospitals should take in preparing themselves against the 'threat of an outbreak' (Commonwealth of Australia 2006a). Alan Dupont, at the University of Sydney, has drawn up hypothetical models which indicate at what point the number of soldiers dying from AIDS in the region could constitute a national security threat to Australia (Dupont 2001). The government also recently conducted a hypothetical infectious disease outbreak emergency, where a 'contaminator' arrived at an airport from an overseas destination, spreading an undiagnosed infectious disease throughout the wider community (Commonwealth of Australia 2006b).

In 1997, the Canadian government set up an electronic surveillance system, the Global Public Health Information Network (GPHIN), which WHO uses to this day as part of the GOARN (see further below) (Grein et al. 2000: 99; Burns 2006: 769). The Canadian government hosted the first G7+ Mexico ministerial meeting which led to the Global Health Security Initiative in 2001, referred to above (Feldbaum and Lee 2004:

23). With the spread of SARS to Toronto in 2003, the Canadian government's understanding of how infectious disease can cause an economy to collapse unless early detection surveillance mechanisms are supported went from a hypothetical scenario to a reality (Aginam 2004: 208; McInnes 2004: 30–35). During the outbreak, the Canadian economy was estimated to have lost $3 billion after SARS was first identified in a Toronto hospital. According to McInnes and Lee (2006: 9), SARS 'demonstrated how policy responses to emerging and re-emerging infectious diseases (ERIDs) can elicit a garrison mentality' in an effort to prevent the spread of infection. Stricter border controls and attempts to regulate migration have been key features in state responses to the spread of infectious disease'. For Canada, SARS also demonstrated that relative geographical isolation was not a strong defence in the face of an epidemic.

Finally, the European Union (EU) has also sought to boost its contribution through treaties and public health surveillance over the last six years (Lee and McInnes 2003: 20). The WHO European Region has discussed the need for a strengthened surveillance capacity for infectious diseases since 2000 so that member states 'have the capacity to detect and respond to epidemics in a timely manner; and to collect the minimum data necessary for action linked to control measures' (WHO 2000b: 1). The EU, like the United States, Australia and Canada, has referred to its public health strategy as a security response representing a 'network for the epidemiological surveillance and control of communicable diseases in the European Union . . . A programme of preparedness and response capacity in the event of attacks involving biological and chemical agents' (Fidler 2004b: 256). The EU has also created an equivalent of the US CDC – the European Centre for Disease Prevention and Control based in Sweden – which monitors the incidence of infectious disease across Eastern and Western Europe. EU members, such as the United Kingdom, have also referred to the risk of disease outbreak in national government policy statements. The British Foreign Office, for example, released a strategy paper in 2003 that described the spread of disease as 'an ill-effect of globalization and a risk to peace and development' (McInnes and Lee 2006: 7).

In late October 2001, anthrax was deliberately released into the United States postal system through envelopes containing a fine powder of anthrax spores. Within a short time twenty-two people were infected, of whom five died. While reference to the use of weaponized biological agents had been made in US government circles as early as 1996 (see above), the release of anthrax soon after the 11 September terrorist attacks in New York and Washington heightened anxiety among states about their vulnerability to such an attack (WHO 2002: 8). The inclusion of bioterrorism into the revised IHR demonstrates the link between bioterrorism and infectious disease that pervades the 'high politics' priorities of many states (Calain 2007: 7).

This section has demonstrated that the risk of infectious disease outbreaks has been increasingly portrayed as a security threat that Western states must take steps to alleviate through their foreign, economic and security policies (McInnes and Lee 2006: 12). At the same time, the increased association of weaponized infectious disease pathogens with traditional security threats (invasion and border integrity) served to heighten interest in global response measures to infectious disease. However, this concern has led to a response that is overtly aimed at protecting Western states from particular infectious disease epidemics, where the investment has been primarily in real-time global disease surveillance, scenario planning, drug stockpiling and vaccine development (Bingham and Hinchliffe 2008: 173–174). The next section will examine how this response is reflected at the global level in the priority that has been accorded to the securitization of particular infectious diseases.

A global response to infectious disease outbreaks

In September 2000, the Millennium Summit was hosted by the United Nations. The Summit formally adopted the Millennium Development Goals (MDGs), which aimed to halve poverty by 2015. Two of the MDGs that directly related to infectious diseases were the reduction of child mortality (goal 4) and goal 6, combating HIV/AIDS, malaria and other diseases (UN 2007). UNICEF has reported success in rates of vaccination for children between 1990 and 2005 (*Lancet* 2007b: 1007), but there remains an urgent need for greater progress in sub-Saharan Africa, Southern Asia, Central Asia and in some areas of Oceania. At the same time, AIDS and malaria still account for high mortality rates in children under the age of five (UN 2007: 15). Evaluations of the success of child mortality reduction also remains mixed, with Murray et al. (2007) reporting that under-5 mortality data used by UNICEF demonstrates that instead of a 67% reduction in deaths as called for by the MDGs, there will only be an actual 27% reduction from 1990 to 2015 (Murray et al. 2007: 1052), while UNICEF maintains that its interpretation of the data refers to an overall reduction in deaths (UN 2007: 15).

Furthermore, a recent report on the progress of the MDGs found that in the area of HIV/AIDS, TB and malaria, the MDG goal to reduce infection and increase treatment by 2015 will not be met (UN 2007: 18–21). In addition, the WHO's Commission on Macroeconomics and Health argued that, to achieve the MDGs, a higher proportion of people needed to have access to safe drinking water and adequate food to combat all preventable disease (Horton 2003: 332–333). The core findings of this Commission were that it was 'the massive amount of disease burden in the world's poorest nations [that] poses a huge threat to global wealth and security' (Stern and Markel 2004: 1474). The second relevant finding was that millions of impoverished people die of preventable and treatable communicable disease because they lack access to basic health care and sanitation and this could be reversed if wealthier nations simply provided poorer countries with funds for basic health care and services (WHO 2001; Sachs and McArthur 2005). However, at present, half of the population in the developing world still lack access to basic sanitation; and the continued lack of access to basic health care services to prevent and treat communicable disease is a theme returned to in the WHO's *2008 World Health Report* (UN 2007: 4; WHO 2008b). This leads us to ask what the securitization of infectious disease has achieved for the majority of people who will be killed by them.

Some argue that in spite of the overall likelihood that the MDGs will not be reached by 2015, the goals represented an attempt to prioritize not just health, but the health of the poor (Lee 2009: 107, 114). Indeed, I would contend that the MDGs were part of a broader institutional attempt by the UN and WHO to link health issues to the realm of 'high politics' through using securitization language as their 'opening' for expanding the global health security agenda from infectious diseases to the broader issue of health inequality.

In 2004, the UN Secretary-General's High Level Panel on Threats, Challenges and Change sought to put forward the case for infectious disease to be considered as a security threat on the grounds that it is unlimited in scope: 'the security of the most affluent State can be held hostage to the ability of the poorest State to contain an emerging disease' (High Level Panel 2004: 14). In essence, failure to invest in the prevention of infectious diseases that affected the majority in poor countries would result in the developed world *also* facing potential insecurity if nothing was done about these preventable deaths: '[T]oday, more than ever before, threats are interrelated and a threat to one is a threat to all' (ibid.).

This message was reinforced by WHO's 2002 Communicable Disease Report: *Global Defence against the Infectious Disease Threat* (Kindhauser 2003). Infectious diseases, WHO argued, may kill the world's poorer citizens – but everyone remains under threat:

The threat posed by infectious disease is now perceived as universally relevant, as the speed and volume of international travel have made an outbreak or epidemic anywhere in the world a potential threat everywhere else. Moreover, the ability of infectious diseases to destabilize societies, so alarmingly demonstrated by AIDS, has brought home the message that local infectious disease problems can have global security implications. (Heymann in WHO 2003: 9)

Furthermore, argued WHO:

Power is unleashed when multiple forces converge, and the infectious disease situation is clearly benefiting. Growing concern over the issue of global health security has resulted in heightened vigilance, better disease intelligence, and strengthened capacity to respond when outbreaks occur. While this trend can be seen as anchored in the enlightened self-interest of nations, the commitment and energy now focused on diseases of the poor are good evidence that humanitarian concerns are likewise shaping the infectious disease situation. (Heymann in WHO 2003: 11)

In the *2007 World Health Report*, WHO argued that 'the public health security of all countries depends on the capacity of each to act effectively and contribute to the security of all' (WHO 2007b: xiii). The WHO defined global public health security in this report as 'the activities required, both proactive and reactive, to minimize vulnerability to acute public health events that endanger the collective health of populations living across geographical regions and international boundaries' (WHO 2007b: ix). WHO was seeking to argue that the health of individuals affected the health of all; but in order to do so, like the High Level Panel, its strategy was to link health equality to national self-interest. Thus, it argued that infectious diseases represented a broader 'threat' that had arisen from public health incapacity in poor states, and therefore required the collective action of the international community (WHO 2007b: xiii).

In this way the MDGs, the UN Secretary-General's High Level Panel and WHO all sought to raise the collective consciousness of states to the security threat posed by infectious diseases, and not just those that primarily concern affluent states (i.e. SARS, pandemic influenza and regional destabilization due to HIV/AIDS). So, in recent years, international organizations have attempted to broaden the scope of what states perceive as a health threat. This effort was based on the premise that even if certain infectious diseases do not threaten wealthier parts of the world at present, they could in the future. Emphasis was placed on the threat to Western nations that would result from their failure to deal with the prevalence of infectious disease in poorer parts of the world. Fidler and Gostin (2008:

15) argue that the benefit of playing the 'security card' in connecting public health and security is that 'biosecurity helps magnify the priority infectious diseases receive in other areas of public health governance, such as development'. For example, the WHO's 2003 *Global Defence against the Infectious Disease Threat* argued that the 'strengthening of global capacity for routine disease surveillance and outbreak response is an essential component of preparedness for a possible attack using biological weapons' (Kindhauser 2003: 17).

In essence, this melding of statist and globalist perspectives (see chapter 1) has sought to persuade Western states that the threat of infectious disease among the world's poor could become a threat to them (Peterson 2006). Emphasis on collective responses to this threat and appeals to enlightened self-interest, it was hoped, would help deliver desperately needed resources (Whitman 2000). For example, David Heymann (2002: 179) argues that simply ensuring enough global investment in epidemiology and laboratory facilities in poorer countries to detect and contain infectious disease outbreaks would produce better surveillance capabilities for all states, which could come into play if and when an outbreak is deliberately caused (i.e. terrorist biological attack), a preoccupation at the 'high politics' level for many Western states.

As I discussed earlier, however, Western states have still tended to focus on the threat that particular infectious diseases may pose to *their* citizens and *their* economies, rather than placing all infectious diseases that afflict the world's poor and vulnerable at the level of 'high politics'. For example, Richard Horton argues that despite Brundtland's efforts to promote health as poverty eradication, the 'strategies to meet the Millennium Development Goals [in the area of health] remain obscure. Political will is fragmented and riven with self-interest' (Horton 2003: 339). *Who* is really protected by global surveillance and infectious disease containment measures (see below) is thus a vital question to ask; as is why a potential influenza pandemic attracts more research funding than tuberculosis when the numbers that die from the latter are much greater right now, and the risk of multidrug-resistant disease means that more will contract tuberculosis and die from it in the immediate future (Aginam 2004). But others challenge this view, and propose that in recent years the UN and WHO's strategy has been successful in achieving levels of global co-operation never previously thought possible due to heightened concerns about health security (Taylor 2004; Weiss and Thakur 2009). It has been argued that the revision of the IHR in 2005 is demonstrative of the fact that, combining globalist and statist concerns, an area of health has been prioritized to a point where the 'rules of the game' have been changed (Fidler 2005). These claims are assessed in the following section.

Revising the International
Health Regulations

On 23 May 2005, the World Health Assembly agreed to revise the IHR, nearly ten years after the first decision to review and revise them in 1996 (WHO 2007b: 12). The revised IHR (2005) came into force in June 2007 and 'provide a legal framework for reporting significant public health risks and events that are identified within national boundaries and for the recommendation of context-specific measures to *stop their international spread*, rather than establishing pre-determined measures aimed at stopping diseases *at international borders* as in the case of IHR (1969)' (emphasis added, WHO 2007b: 12).

The blueprint for the WHO's IHR dates back to 1851 when a cholera epidemic swept through Europe and caused immense panic in cities (McNeill 1998; Lee and Dodgson 2003; Harrison 2004). The epidemic had a devastating effect on economic and political stability in many European capitals and their surrounds. People and exports were quarantined for lengthy periods, while residents fled cities in fear of contracting the disease. These events led to the first multilateral co-operation in the area of public health at the International Sanitary Conference held in Paris in 1851. This conference, led by France, attempted to create and then promote collective adherence to measures that would 'protect Europe from disease importations and [yet] to lessen the burden quarantine placed on international trade' (Fidler 1999: 28). However, there was a clash between Britain's emphasis on each state introducing public health reform and sanitary measures, and European countries (particularly along the Mediterranean coast) who argued that such measures were not affordable (Fidler 1999: 32). More to the point, several European countries, including France, Italy and Spain, argued that it was Britain's imperial reach that was causing 'Asiatic' diseases such as cholera to spread through their states and therefore strict quarantine measures was the best solution to protect themselves (McNeill 1998; Harrison 2004). This argument continued up until the turn of the century and European states continued to dominate the International Sanitary Conferences (1892, 1893, 1894 and 1897) without stamping out cholera or yellow fever (there were disease epidemics of both in Europe in the late 1800s) the Convention instrument also covered bubonic plague (Fidler 1999: 29–30). Thus, there was little real progress in international health co-operation until 1903 (Goodman 1971: 36–42; McNeill 1998: 281; Fidler 2005).

The 1903 Convention consolidated the four conventions from the previous conferences and set out specific implementation guidelines. The new Convention primarily concerned cholera and the plague, with only a brief mention of the threat of yellow fever. The 1903 Convention contained 184 articles in ten chapters and was signed by twenty countries, with sixteen having ratified it by 1907. The chapters dealt with pilgrims travelling to and from Mecca (which was believed to be linked to epidemics of cholera and the plague); the International Sanitary Councils of Alexandria, Constantinople and Tangier; the Suez Canal, Red Sea and Persian Gulf; it also included quarantine measures for trade and migrant arrivals, as well as epidemiological notification procedures (Goodman 1971: 70). There were classifications allocated for ship inspections, period of observations and 'deratization' requirements.[7]

The 1903 International Sanitary Convention therefore represented a new level of international co-operation in relation to health matters. Though the purpose was again largely to protect trade and migration paths, the agreement that all affected members should undertake 'collective' interventions and procedures in the event of an outbreak of cholera, plague or yellow fever reflected the increasing seriousness with which participating states treated the threat that infectious disease could pose to trade. Watts (1997), McNeill (1998), Harrison (2004) and Diamond (2005) argue that increased scientific knowledge about microbes and the conditions that enabled their spread also played a key role in persuading governments of the value of implementing these new measures.

Between 1903 and the establishment of WHO there were few amendments to the 1903 Convention. Therefore, by the time WHO's Constitution came into force in 1948, newly emerged states and those with experience of the 1903 Convention were ready to support a universal body to represent 'every conceivable element in the field of health' (Pannenborg 1979: 184). The WHO was intended as a new form of international governance in the area of health that would serve to protect states from the potential harms caused by ill health (see chapter 2). This created a desire for consensus in all WHO operations, based on the calculation that states would realize that, whenever they sought to opt out of collective measures that would protect the health of their citizens, they would create undue risk to their own economic and social stability. Pannenborg (1979) argues that this was best reflected by the unanimous adoption of the International Sanitary Conventions by the World Health Assembly in 1951, renamed the International Sanitary Regulations. Later, in 1969, WHO would rename them the International Health Regulations (IHR) and while little of the IHR would be revised until 2005, it was promoted as the best example of 'infectious disease diplomacy' between countries (WHO 2002: 2). However, in practice, the IHR suffered from 'patchy compliance among WHO member states' (WHO 2007b: 11). Paradoxically though, states did not seek limits or restraints to WHO's power in this area, nor did they seek the dissolution of the IHR. Ironically, the patchy compliance and WHO's own reluctance to enforce the IHRs contributed to their durability and universal acceptance (Taylor 1992).

The IHR (1951–2005) obliged member states to notify WHO of cholera, plague and yellow fever outbreaks in their territory, and to follow health-related rules for international trade and travel. Requirements included vaccination of possible carriers, disinfection of ships and aircraft, as well as quarantine measures at airports and seaports in affected areas. There were separate protocols on notification for outbreaks of relapsing fever, smallpox and typhus. In 1995, WHO headquarters sought substantial revision to the IHR, listing five key constraints that were hampering the organization's response to infectious disease outbreaks. First, the IHR were limited in its coverage. Only three diseases were listed in the regulations, yet WHO had identified at least '40 diseases that were unknown a generation ago' (WHO 2007b: x); and by the 1990s, there had been a proliferation of quite virulent infectious diseases, such as the haemorrhagic fevers, that WHO argued required states to provide an immediate alert to ensure strict quarantine and verification regulations. Second, WHO could not insist that an affected government notify them of an outbreak under the IHR, particularly if the outbreak involved a disease that was not covered by the IHR. Third, there were no procedures to guide collaboration between WHO and the affected country in the containment of disease. Fourth, the only incentive encouraging compliance with notification procedures was a negative one, i.e. the deterrent effect if a country thought they would get caught for non-compliance. WHO argued this form of compliance was too risky in the situations where countries might delay notification in the hope that they could avoid having to notify WHO. Important time could be lost as the disease travelled across borders without any precautions in place to prevent or contain its spread. Finally, there were no risk-specific measures or global surveillance in place to prevent and trace the spread of disease (WHO 2002: 3).

A number of events led WHO to issue its call for a revision of the IHR in 1995. The Cold War had ended six years earlier, ostensibly improving the chances of consensus in the WHA. The risk of new emerging infectious diseases (EID) and re-emerging infectious diseases (REID) was considered to pose new dangers to populations with little immunity or none to diseases for which there might be no known prevention or cure. Finally, WHO argued, it was no longer possible for states to deal with infectious disease outbreaks individually (Fidler et al. 1997). The increased rate of travel and trade associated with globalization (Lee 2003) raised concerns about the speed at which a new infectious disease could travel via a human, water or food host to another country before effective containment measures could be put in place. At the same time, the end of the Cold War raised concerns about the possibility of, for example, dilapidated laboratories in Eastern Europe 'misplacing' their biological agent stockpile, which could be used by terrorists against civilian populations through underground rail systems or via water supply systems (Garrett 2001).

On top of all of this, an outbreak of plague in India in 1994 proved that neither WHO nor the IHR had the capacity to deliver responses that could deal with a health crisis while protecting states from negative economic repercussions (Carvalho and Zacher 2001: 252–255). When India notified WHO of a suspected bubonic plague outbreak, panic ensued, with trade and travel embargoes placed on India that resulted in economic losses of $1.7 billion. After the event, WHO concluded that the international response had included 'unnecessary countermeasures' (WHO 2002: 3). The story began in September 1994 when seven people with pneumonia-like symptoms were hospitalized in Surat Civil Hospital, Gujarat. Before tests on those hospitalized had been concluded the Indian government notified the public of a suspected plague outbreak (Cash and Narasimhan 2000: 1360). In accordance with IHR, the Indian Ministry of Health formally notified WHO, examined persons leaving the country with flu-like symptoms and fumigated cargo from all ports against rodent infestation (Cash and Narasimhan 2000: 1361). In addition, individuals with suspected infection were kept in quarantine and all schools were closed. However, neither WHO nor the Indian government was able to control the immense panic that ensued after the Indian government's public notice. Approximately 500,000 people fled Surat, including essential health workers (Cash and Narasimhan 2000: 1361; Enemark 2007: 129). This mass flight only increased concerns that the disease might spread into other Indian states and even neighbouring countries.

The global reaction to the plague outbreak in India demonstrated two things: first, that WHO had little control over how states followed the disease alert and response measures under the existing IHR; second, states would be even more reluctant to notify WHO about disease outbreaks in light of India's experience (WHO 2002: 3). After India, states recognized that the mismanagement of outbreaks could have serious negative effects on economic and political stability, making them more receptive to the idea of revising the IHR (WHO 2002; Heymann 2003). But it was not enough to secure consensus on what the revised IHR should look like (e.g. Taylor 1997; Frenk et al. 2001).

David Fidler has been a prominent advocate of the idea that the IHR revisions marked a shift away from the traditional emphasis on the state as the sole primary actor to respond to an infectious disease outbreak.

Fidler (2004c, 2005, 2007b) refers to the outbreak of SARS – which origi-nated in Guangdong province, China, in November 2002 – as the catalyst for progress in the IHR revisions. China at first attempted to keep secret the outbreak of an unknown but serious and fatal pneumonia (Kimball 2006: 45). Doctors from Guangzhou eventually alerted the world to the disease in February 2003, but by then, a very ill 62-year-old SARS-infected phy-sician had travelled from Guangzhou to Hong Kong, where he succumbed to the illness. It appears that this doctor was the 'index' case, or first case linked to the spread of the infection to other states, as his stay at a hotel in Hong Kong was linked to the disease spreading among hotel guests who travelled on to Singapore, Taiwan, Vietnam and Canada (Kimball 2006: 47). WHO's effort to co-ordinate international laboratory collaboration led to the identification of the virus within one month and the implementation of quarantine measures, including travel warnings, 'stand down' measures in hospitals, and checking the body temperature of all travellers at airports in the affected regions (Kimball 2006; WHO 2007b).

The swift international response to the outbreak represented a moment, Fidler argues (2004a), of 'good governance' which served to galvanize state support for what had been, until then, a painfully slow eight-year discussion of IHR revisions. SARS demonstrated a need for the capacity and co-operation of different public and private laboratories, public health officials and WHO to work on disease diagnosis and quarantine alerts. The threat posed by newly emerging infectious diseases was demonstrated by the SARS outbreak, prompting faster consensus on the need for global infectious disease control measures – where a variety of actors (not just states) engaged in disease surveillance and notification (Heymann 2005; Kimball 2006). Global control measures would now require a 'vertical and horizontal process' (Fidler 2004a: 800) where states, international organi-zations, NGOs, public health officials and even pharmaceutical companies had to work together on infectious disease control.

Most crucial was the role played by the Global Outbreak Alert and Response Network in the case of SARS. GOARN was created at a time when delays in the IHR revisions were frustrating WHO (Davies 2008). The argument made was that, in the meantime, there needed to be a global surveillance network which could gather outbreak reports from across the world on a 24-hour, 7 days a week basis in order to manage outbreak veri-fication and response (WHO 2002: 23). This led to the creation in 1997 of the first global infectious disease surveillance system, the Global Public Health Information Network. The GPHIN, funded entirely by the Canadian government, is a web-based electronic system that scans the worldwide web to identify suspected outbreaks (Burns 2006: 769). Between 2000 and 2002, WHO lobbied for the creation of GOARN, which would receive GPHIN alerts, seek state outbreak verification, and send fieldwork response teams to the outbreak site if the state requested WHO's assistance (WHO 2002: 3). For its part, the GOARN was to 'improve epidemic disease control by informing key public health professionals about confirmed and unconfirmed outbreaks of international public health importance' (Grein et al. 2000: 97).

In the case of SARS, the Chinese government was initially reluctant to notify WHO of the rate of infection, but at the same time unable to control the information flow because alternative actors independently contacted WHO via GOARN (Fidler 2004c; Kimball 2006). The fact that actors such as NGOs, the media, and health staff at hospitals contacted WHO – and did so independent of the Chinese government – affirmed WHO's authority in the containment of infectious disease on behalf of the global community and highlighted a key feature of globalization: the uncontrollable flow of information (Davies 2008). Likewise, the fact that all SARS-affected states (except China) proceeded to co-operate and notify WHO of their outbreaks, even when the organization started to release travel notifications and public statements about SARS-infected zones, has been represented as an important shift in WHO's authority (Heymann and Rodier 2004). In this case, it is apparent that the threat of an infectious disease outbreak was considered more important than protecting sovereign control of information. None of the affected states was legally obliged or coerced to inform WHO, because the old IHR had no jurisdiction over SARS, but the ramifications of not co-operating with WHO trumped efforts to deal with it internally as key groups and individuals sought WHO's assistance (Taylor 2004: 501; Rodier in Burns 2006).

Allyn Taylor (2004: 501) has argued that the link of health to global security has given it a central place in international relations – and in turn – global governance. This link has enabled the use of international law to create new international health commitments, such as the revised IHR (see below), and Taylor (2004) argues, opens a 'Pandora's box' of possibilities for WHO to elevate its place in international affairs. The revised IHR were unanimously passed by the WHA on 23 May 2005. Fidler (2004c: 127–128) argues that WHO's success was largely due to the post-SARS realization that 'international cooperation on infectious diseases required a permanent, central international organization'. Furthermore, SARS led to a realization for states that:

[I]n a globalized world, states need to give public health more attention and resources. Such political concern for public health can play a significant role in addressing threats from globalizing diseases . . . The need for such political commitment cut across the spectrum of states in the international system, implicating rich and poor countries, liberal states and authoritarian regimes. (Fidler 2004c: 149)

Meanwhile, Calain argued that the revised IHR (which came into force in June 2007) would be more influential than its precursor because '(1) the broader scope of health events under [its] consideration, (2) a more active and better defined role for WHO in the response phase, and (3) more flexible mechanisms for WHO to circulate information critical to control public health threats (including information from non-official sources or about non-compliant state parties)' (2007: 5). Some in WHO argued that WHA consensus to draft IHR revisions after SARS demonstrated a collective understanding that 'as long as national capacities are weak, international mechanisms for outbreak alert and response will be needed' (Heymann and Rodier 2004: 173). Cathy Roth argues that there 'is no single institution or agency that has all the capacity to approach and tackle such emergencies. WHO is able to achieve the goals of its strategic approach by bringing partners together to focus and coordinate global responses' (Roth 2006: 101).

The revised IHR defines disease of concern to IHR as more broadly 'an illness or medical condition, irrespective of origin or source, that presents or could present significant harm to humans'.[8] A disease 'event' now requires a response from WHO if it signified 'a manifestation of disease or an occurrence that creates a potential for disease'. Finally, a 'public health risk' could be identified, and thus require WHO intervention, when the 'likelihood of an event that may affect adversely the health of human populations, with an emphasis on one which may spread internationally or may present a serious or direct danger' (WHO 2005a). WHO has described the revised IHR as a 'living international legal instrument which . . . will require States Parties and WHO to take concrete, often daily actions to prevent, protect against, control and provide public health responses to the international spread of disease' (WHO 2005a). The late WHO Director-General, Dr Lee Jong-Wook, argued that the WHA's acceptance of the revised IHR was not just a major step for international health but also recognition 'that diseases do not respect national boundaries' (WHO 2005b).

The understandable efforts by states to protect their economy, political stability and society from the fear generated by an infectious disease outbreak by keeping it quiet is now counterbalanced by the legal obligation to notify WHO and follow the 'decision instrument' drawn up by WHO for ascertaining whether the situation constitutes a public health emergency of international concern (PHEIC). Under Annex 2 of the IHR, a PHEIC calls on states and non-state actors (such as those run by disease surveillance networks like ProMED or humanitarian agencies on the ground) to report public health risks that may cause the international spread of disease, even if the outbreak is outside their territory. WHO is to be instantly notified via GOARN under the PHEIC mechanism, and the Emergency Committee can 'make temporary recommendations in order to prevent or reduce the international spread of disease and to minimize interference with international traffic' (WHO 2005a). The evolution of the IHR revisions indicates that WHO has succeeded in arguing that the urgency of infectious disease requires new and innovative forms of global health governance. The claim that the threat of an infectious disease outbreak is so great that it necessitates a response beyond sovereign states had led to the argument that sovereignty must come second to epidemic control (WHO 2005b). Such an argument demonstrates that the securitization of health has, at least within this area, been successful (Zacher 2007). Unanimous agreement to the revised IHR demonstrates that states have responded to WHO's call for recognition of the existential threat that infectious disease poses and the idea that, if states do not recognize the importance of the threat, WHO should have the capacity under GOARN to respond to alerts provided by actors, including non-state actors, and demand state verification of an outbreak. Ostensibly, this is the product of the securitization of infectious disease: societies need protection from infectious disease to survive and therefore must suspend prevailing sovereignty norms to reduce the threat (Buzan et al. 1998b: 36). The statist perspective has blended with the globalist perspective to produce a situation where a health issue is deemed (in theory at least) to be so important for the protection of all states that the reluctance of one state to co-operate in this global surveillance regime should not prevent the capacity of WHO and other states to protect their citizens. Traditionally, states have decided what constitutes a threat to their citizens, yet technically, under GOARN and the revised IHR, WHO can determine what constitutes a threat, and even what action the state needs to take to reduce it. This level of responsibility bestowed on WHO has not only made it a more powerful actor, but also a securitizing actor. It may be possible that the newly emerging threat of infectious diseases has brought about a new understanding of which actor is best placed to provide security (Buzan et al. 1998b: 36–39).

However, there are a number of unresolved problems that should give us cause for concern. First, from a practical point of view, the revised IHR still requires verification from the state where the outbreak is located before WHO can issue an international alert or respond with containment measures. Although GOARN may be alerted by actors other than states in the advent of an infectious disease outbreak, the responsibility for verifying an outbreak still rests with the affected state. Therefore, the sovereign state remains a crucial actor that both the revised IHR and GOARN must defer to before they can activate disease containment measures.

Second, Calain argues that 'misperceptions about the rationale for global surveillance generated by such conflicts of interest or blurred agendas will probably fuel further concerns about their sovereignty among Member States when it comes to enacting the revised IHR' (2007: 9). In essence, arguments that the revised IHR heralds the supremacy of global governance over sovereign states in the area of infectious diseases might be premature. Developing states may be reluctant to cede their sovereignty for fear of WHO serving as a Trojan horse for external interference in their domestic affairs (Mack 2006; Calain 2007). Essentially, global governance cannot be 'top-down' – it needs the co-operation and engagement of all actors, not just Western governments seeking to protect themselves from the outbreaks they deem most likely to reach their shores. The concern is that, due to the financial support that Western states have provided for notification procedures, they will be able to use WHO to pressure developing states to verify outbreak alerts that concern their interests rather than treating all disease outbreaks with the same level of concern. The consequence, Calain (2007: 8) argues, could be that states most in need of assistance with disease containment measures may actually increase their resistance to external efforts to manage outbreaks in their territory. For example, we have seen this since 2005 with Indonesia attempting to restrict WHO's access to H5N1 human infection specimens collected from Indonesian citizens. The Indonesian government contends that the specimens are state owned and not to be accessed or shared by WHO. Their concern is that, if WHO shares the virus on its influenza network, and a Western pharmaceutical company develops an H5N1 vaccine from the sample, Indonesia would have to buy back the vaccine at an exorbitant price under the present patent and intellectual property arrangements (Supari 2008; see chapter 7).

Third, as Peterson (2006) argues, the securitization discourse surrounding infectious disease fails to fully address the fact that, unless an infectious disease outbreak poses a direct threat to Western states' national security, very few of them will treat such disease outbreaks seriously. In short, donor funds will only flow to those diseases that pose a threat to the West. This is of vital concern as implementing the revised IHR and GOARN relies on continued donor interest (Peterson 2006: 46). Therefore, maintaining the interest of Western states in infectious diseases could lead to continued investments in GOARN, drug research and vaccine development with the purpose of protecting these states from the threat of a disease outbreak; but can 'global' co-operation be expected if there is little investment in structures that will assist developing states to build their basic public health capacity? Indeed, it has been acknowledged by WHO that

GOARN is 'primarily targeted at developing states' (WHO 2000). As David Fidler and Lawrence Gostin (2006) acknowledge, while the IHR revisions emphasize health system strengthening, there has been no extra donor state funding attached to states achieving the IHR revision benchmarks. The danger is that, without incentives, including substantial support for capacity-building in the public health systems of developing states, progress will be difficult to achieve (for example) in the area of pandemic preparedness. In addition, calling on states to reorganize their health priorities in order to satisfy international demands for improved surveillance and verification overlooks the fact that some states have other competing health priorities that pose a more serious and immediate threat to their populations than the possible outbreak of pandemic influenza or a bioterrorist attack, as discussed at the beginning of this chapter.

Conclusion

The elevation of infectious disease from a public health concern to a global security concern, through mechanisms such as the revised IHR and GOARN, has led some to herald the beginning of the 'post-Westphalian state' (Fidler 2003c). In the Westphalian era, 'public health was premised on the principle that states constituted the only legitimate actors for governance purposes' (Fidler 2003c: 488). The participation of non-state actors during the 1990s, to the point where WHO was able to set up a mechanism such as GOARN, meant that there was less need for states to inform the international community of a disease outbreak and represented a major break from the previous reliance on states for disease outbreak notification. However, on closer inspection, it is not entirely clear that this means the state is needed less in formulating a disease containment strategy in the face of a pandemic, or that Western states have accepted the practice of securitization for all infectious diseases, not just those that they fear reaching their shores.

Despite significant progress towards globalized responses to infectious diseases, the state still has the primary role and final jurisdiction (Fidler 2007b). Furthermore, while Western states consider infectious diseases to be a concern of 'high politics' (though only to the extent that it may be likely to threaten them), WHO has attempted (with little success) to highlight the wider threat presented by communicable diseases more generally that afflict the poorer parts of the world. Mechanisms such as GOARN and the revised IHR could, ostensibly, improve individual safety from disease outbreaks regardless of where they occur. But this will not happen if states only see these mechanisms as tools of containment for protecting themselves from virulent infectious diseases (Davies 2008). To date, the consequence of bringing infectious disease to the realm of 'high politics' has been that only particular diseases have been admitted and many of those that exact the highest morbidity and mortality in the world's poorest places have been excluded and, even, de-emphasized.

7 HEALTH AS A BUSINESS

As has been made apparent in earlier chapters there is a pervasive tension in the contemporary global politics of health in ensuring that particular health issues receive the attention from states that they deserve by placing them in the realm of 'high politics' through securitization and other mechanisms, without compromising the needs and rights of individuals and communities, especially the most vulnerable. The proliferation of non-state actors has widened the number of those interested and engaged with health issues, and broadened the scope of global engagement, but it has not resolved this underlying tension. The final set of issues discussed in this book is one that has not lacked attention in the last decade or so from global health actors. I label this area the international political economy of health (IPEH). IPEH research in both the Public Health and International Relations disciplines has expanded in recent years to highlight a number of health issues that have direct relevance to broader international concerns – from the most talked-about area of pharmaceutical trade and patents, through to the debate about the privatization of health care sectors in low- and middle-income countries, the global effects of the migration of health workers from low-income to high-income countries and the role of private companies in exporting addictive substances such as tobacco to low-income countries that have little or no regulations on such sales.

In this chapter, I will briefly examine four critical issues relating to IPEH. Two of these issues – access to prescription medicines and health tourism – have attracted much attention in the fields of public health, economics, anthropology, law, philosophy and politics. The other two – offshore clinical trials and vaccine research – have received less multidisciplinary attention but are, I argue, important issues to examine in order to gain a clear picture of how IPEH operates at the local, international and global levels.

As I noted in the introduction, the thirty OECD countries make up less than 20% of the world's population but spend 90% of the world's resources on health (WHO 2007a: 19). Essentially, WHO argues, this means that 'richer countries with smaller populations and lower disease burdens use more health resources than poorer countries with larger populations and higher disease burdens' (WHO 2007a: 19). Because IPEH takes economics as its starting point, the perspectives differ somewhat from the globalist and statist approaches identified in chapter 1 though the tensions made apparent by thinking about the global politics of health in statist and globalist terms are evident in this domain as well. Thus, the main perspectives in IPEH are what I term the utilitarian approach and a health equity approach. The health equity approach – which shares much in common with the Critical Security Studies perspective – seeks to address health inequalities, which it says exist due to a collective failure to 'go beyond health achievement and the capability to achieve public health' (Sen 2004: 24). This approach, in common with the globalist perspective, prioritizes the rights and needs of individuals. In contrast, the utilitarian approach seeks to provide a path to affordable health care for as many people as possible in a way that is financially sustainable and cost-effective – for this approach 'the objective should be to identify those aspects of quality which will maximize effectiveness at least cost while promoting the financial sustainability of the health service' (Wouters 1991: 269). The utilitarian approach seeks a cost-effective and sustainable approach to health care delivery. However, while utilitarians may not believe that health care delivery is always best managed by the state, they subscribe to the statist view that the state plays a crucial stabilizing role in health politics – allowing the conditions for affordable health care to be available to the greatest number of people. According to the utilitarian approach, access to health care needs to be determined by cost-effectiveness analysis (CEA).[1] To achieve this goal, the utilitarian approach has produced the disability-adjusted life years or DALYs (see chapter 2) and the quality-adjusted life years or QALYs (Culyer and Wagstaff 1993).[2] The differences between the health equity and utilitarian approaches revolve around a debate concerning how best to deliver health care in a world of scarce resources and multiple demands for those resources; again, this is a debate that is not dissimilar to the statist and globalist perspective.

In this chapter, I will highlight how these competing approaches offer different answers to questions about access to prescription medicines, offshore clinical trials, vaccine delivery and health tourism. I will argue that the core concern about *how* to deliver the best care to individuals is always adjacent to contention about *who* should be delivering this care and the resources that ought to be committed. What is significant about the area of IPEH is that, in an era characterized by global health governance, the actors who sometimes have the most direct influence on the health of individuals are not states or international organizations such as WHO and the World Bank. I do not for a moment suggest that these actors are unimportant, as demonstrated by the fact that their failure at times to take the lead in this and in a committee to continued health inequity (as discussed in chapter 2). But private companies and philanthropic foundations have become crucial actors in the IPEH, shaping advocacy, innovation and health outcomes that have a direct effect on the health of individuals (Leach et al. 2005: 107). Each of the four areas I discuss in this chapter involve private organizations playing a large role in determining the type and level of health care delivery available in low- and middle-income countries. In each case, the key theme is the increasingly important relationship between the developing state and private actors, which can work for either good or bad health outcomes.

The first issue discussed in this chapter is the debate concerning access to prescription medicines, in particular the debate about access to patent medicines that has arisen since the Trade-Related Aspects of Intellectual Property Rights (TRIPS) agreement in 1994. I will identify how the health equity and utilitarian approaches offer different accounts of the responsibility that pharmaceutical companies bear for access to medicines.

The second issue is offshore clinical trials. Here again, we see the important role of pharmaceutical companies in influencing health care delivery through their efforts to promote low-cost research and development (R&D) trials in low- and middle-income countries. R&D trials in low-income states can be conducted relatively cheaply and can often relieve strained health care systems by providing health checks as *quid pro quo* for clinical trials. The consequences, however, range from states avoiding the responsibility to provide health care to their citizens without the support of pharmaceutical companies to individuals being vulnerable to aggressive campaigning by pharmaceutical companies wanting to conduct controversial placebo trials and low-cost testing in an environment with markedly reduced regulatory and ethical scrutiny (Melrose 1982; Shah 2006). Proponents argue that, despite the limited short-term benefits that offshore clinical testing provides for developing countries, it is vital for ensuring continued low-cost R&D, which will improve the availability of drugs in low- and middle-income countries (Freeman 2006). Others, however, argue that offshore clinical trials exploit poor people's need for low-cost health care (Angell 2004). The increased use of offshore clinical trials is widening the discussion about the role and responsibility of pharmaceutical companies, whose status as key actors in the delivery of health care has received comparatively little attention to date.

The chapter then discusses vaccine programmes, in particular, the rising number of projects devoted to vaccination against diseases such as malaria and the search for a HIV vaccine. Again, the core actors driving the vaccination agenda are non-state actors such as the Gates Foundation and pharmaceutical companies such as GlaxoSmithKline. While these activities are commendable and will undoubtedly save lives, we see contention between health equity advocates and utilitarians. Some question whether a malarial vaccine, for example, is the 'magic bullet' for stemming the massive loss of life and health in countries racked by malaria or if, in fact, the key lies in programmes to improve public health systems. Again, as in the case of offshore clinical trials, the focus of private organizations is on the potential for medical innovation with relatively little consideration of how health systems will improve as a result of vaccine development. There are also important issues surrounding the long-term sustainability of these programmes.

The fourth and final area, health tourism, raises a number of questions about state investment in affordable health care and the economic benefits that derive from building state-of-the-art capabilities and procedures for people who, ironically, are unable to afford such treatment in their own states. The idea of low- and middle-income countries providing cosmetic surgery and heart, orthopaedic and transplant operations for those from high-income countries who cannot access such treatment in their own home country contrasts strikingly with the fact that the majority of those in the country where these 'health tourism' services are provided cannot access this care themselves. The ramifications range from philosophical questions about whether states should be encouraging the privatization of specialist health care over the provision of basic affordable access for their own citizens, to the practical problem of highly skilled health workers deserting public clinics and hospitals for the more lucrative private sphere.

The primary focus in each of these sections will be to draw out the tensions between the two different philosophies of health equity and utilitarianism in how they seek to allocate economic resources to strengthen world health. Health equity is animated by the idea that health is a human right and that the state has a responsibility to provide health care. In contrast, the utilitarian position proposes that the market is the best distributor of scarce health goods and the state's role is limited to protecting the market. From their perspective, health treatment is conditional on what can be provided in an economically sustainable fashion and this is the extent of the state's duty to its citizens. The overall purpose of this chapter is to reveal that both approaches need to deal with the rise of private actors that pull or push the state's role in health provision, whether it is through states having to accommodate pharmaceutical costs in their yearly health budget or privatizing certain hospitals to accommodate rising consumerist demands. Both approaches face tension in the need for the state to regulate health access, even at a minimum level, while operating in an economic environment characterized by private actors. The key question that this chapter seeks to explore is whether the state can best develop a health system that will benefit its citizens through resituating itself in the core business of health.

Access to essential drugs

In 1977, WHO defined the term 'essential medicines' as 'those drugs that satisfy the healthcare needs of the majority of the population and that should therefore be available at all times, in adequate amounts and appropriate dosage forms and at a price that individuals and the community can afford' (Lush 2004: 3). WHO published a list of 208 essential drugs in the same year, identifying these as the drugs that all countries should prioritize in their national drug distribution system (Lush 2004: 3). WHO determined what drugs should be placed on this list (some generic and some that are not) by reference to four criteria: rational selection (drug best able to treat widest range of afflictions); affordable prices; sustainable and adequate financing; and a reliable health care and supply system (WHO-WTO 2002: 214). Since 1975, the Essential Drugs List has led to two-thirds of the world having regular access to essential medicines – up from just under one-half when the initiative began (Leach et al. 2005: 3). The Drugs List has achieved this thanks to two main factors: first, the widespread dissemination of this list. The list itself created a powerful normative case for the drugs to be provided at an affordable cost. Second, the system itself has led to better regulation, better production, usage control and lower prices (Lush 2004: 4). However, a broader perspective highlights other factors which paint a less rosy picture. Not least, population growth means that access has not remained constant and income level still greatly affects access to essential medicines (Leach et al. 2005: 3). Approximately 80% of the world's population lives without access to essential medicines, with India and Africa accounting for 53% of those living without access to essential medicines (ibid.). Furthermore, between 50% and 90% of the cost of drugs is paid for as an out-of-pocket expense – this means that poor households bear the highest cost burden for essential medicines (WHO-WTO 2002: 215; Lush 2004: 5).

Health equity advocates argue that WHO and the states that house big pharmaceutical companies (the United States, Japan, Switzerland and the United Kingdom are home to the top ten pharmaceutical companies) should place pressure on those companies to realize their moral duty to provide essential drugs at more reasonable prices. In addition, they argue that these governments should increase their financial aid in order to assist low-income countries in creating a larger public sector budget to pay for essential medicines (Barry and Raworth 2002; Ford 2004; Preker 2004; Leach et al. 2005). The contrasting utilitarian argument holds that the high cost burden being borne by poor households is due to the overprescription of medicines in low-income countries, which is due to poor health systems that are unable to recommend and monitor appropriate drug intake (Attaran and Gillespie-White 2001; Resnik 2001; Lippert 2002; Lush 2004;[3] Attaran and Granville 2004).

Before 2001, some of the most innovative drug therapies for illnesses such as malaria, TB and HIV were not available on the Essential Drugs List due to their inability to meet WHO's four criteria. Then in 2001, WHO removed the low-cost criterion for placing drugs on the List; this led to antiretrovirals for HIV treatment and therapy for drug-resistant tuberculosis making the List for the first time. Debate continues about whether removing the cost criterion addresses the wider problems associated with ensuring that new and innovative therapies are available to the poor – who often have most need for these drugs and at the same time are least likely to be able to afford them (Ford 2004: 138; Leach et al. 2005: 106–107). What continues to concern advocates for a broader criterion on essential drug access, which would widen the List still further, is that putting anti-retrovirals or TB drugs on the List does not automatically mean that the populations most in need of these drugs will be able to afford them (Usdin 2007: 54). Nor does widening the term 'essential' mean that the problems associated with poorly funded health care systems will be addressed – people need to be able to afford a visit to the doctor before they can even start thinking about what drug they can or cannot afford (Attaran and Granville 2004; Curci and Vittori 2004; Ford 2004).

Healthy equity advocates argue that the problem with access to medicines stems from the unwillingness of pharmaceutical companies to reduce costs and allow production of generic (unbranded) equivalents (*Lancet* 2002: 885; Vande Walle and Ponsaers 2006: 368). In contrast, utilitarians maintain that the access problem is caused by an environment where there is ineffective health care system delivery, which makes the use of new treatments potentially dangerous. Moreover, they argue that profits are important to stimulate and fund future research (Resnik 2001; Attaran and Granville 2004). As this section unfolds, it will become clear that both approaches have merit. On the one hand, generic production would go a long way to reducing the high cost burden that the world's poor have to bear for access to essential drugs (two-thirds in the developing world compared to one-fifth in the developed world pay out of pocket for essential drugs; Lush 2004: 6). On the other hand, there is also a valid concern that in countries where access to qualified health professionals is limited, greater drug affordability may also increase the risk of drug abuse through inappropriate self-medication. This poses a real risk of secondary illnesses and, in the case of TB, HIV, respiratory illnesses and malaria, increased drug resistance. Increased drug resistance then creates additional problems for the wider population (Shadlen 2007). These issues came to a head with the TRIPS agreement at the Uruguay Round of the GATT which led to the creation of the World Trade Organization (WTO).

TRIPS was created to ensure that products developed by private companies would remain under the 'ownership' of that company for a specific period – ensuring that cheaper copies could not be made and sold. In relation to health, TRIPS was primarily intended to protect pharmaceutical companies by expecting all signatory countries to accept and comply with drug patents for a twenty-year period (Kumaranayake 2006: 332). Under the agreement, products created before 1 January 1995 were exempted, but products created after that date cannot be produced generically until the twenty-year patent expires. All countries that are signatories to TRIPS were expected to put regulations in place by 2006 that would prevent domestic companies producing generic forms of patented pharmaceuticals. In response to the advent of pharmaceutical patents in countries such as India and Brazil, where generic production has been high, there would now be 'fair return for costly innovation' for the mainly Western pharmaceutical companies that created these drugs (Scherer 2004: 1141).

Like the industry itself, the introduction of patents for pharmaceuticals is relatively new. The pharmaceutical industry did not really take off as a high-profit industry until after World War II (von Braun and Pugatch 2005: 600) and, in the key countries where the pharmaceutical industry exists, patents did not arrive until the 1960s (Nogues 1993: 26). In 1999, the pharmaceutical industry was recorded as having one of, if not the, highest profit margins of 30% compared to the majority of other industries which sat between 5% and 10% (Resnik 2001: 13). In terms of R&D expenditure, Resnik argues that the annual cost of pharmaceutical R&D in the United States alone is around $26.4 billion or more than 60% of total biomedical R&D funding spent in the country (2001: 14). This is compared to 'only' $14 billion which the companies spend on marketing (Resnik 2001: 14). It should be noted, though, that Resnik's figures come from the Pharmaceutical Research and Manufacturing Association. Others argue that independent analysis has shown that marketing costs for the pharmaceutical industry are as high as 30% of their total expenditure, compared to 12% expended on R&D, and in the United States, where nearly two-thirds of the global pharmaceutical industry is housed, pharmaceuticals are taxed at a lower rate than other industries (an 8–10% difference) (Benatar 2003: 69). In addition, the pharmaceutical industry does not make profits from diseases that need treatment in India and Africa. Instead, the bulk of their profit is made in developed countries (Schuklenk 2003: 65).

The utilitarian case therefore rests on two key assumptions. First, the argument is that the pharmaceutical industry may have higher than average profits, but this is necessary to cover the costly R&D. Second, protection for the pharmaceutical industry is necessary because of the important humanitarian role that it plays in creating drugs, a role that is abused by countries that do not respect patent protection (Resnik 2001: 14). However, the cost of R&D bears little relationship to the profit and marketing expenditure of 'Big Pharma'. Moreover, only 5% of the total money spent worldwide on medical R&D is for diseases that primarily affect developing countries, challenging Resnik's defence of pharmaceutical companies as good humanitarians (Shuklenk 2003). Of the 1,395 drugs developed and approved between 1975 and 1999, only thirteen were for tropical diseases, including tuberculosis and malaria (Pollock and Price 2003: 571). Industrial countries presently hold 97% of patents worldwide and 80% of the patent licences granted to developing countries still belong to industrial countries (ibid.).

The argument that generic competition impacts on the ability of pharmaceutical companies to recoup expenses on R&D has also come under criticism. Loff and Heywood (2002: 626) argue that generic production actually has little financial impact on the profits of big pharmaceutical companies. For example, GlaxoSmithKline actually achieved a 15% increase in profit between 2000 and 2001, after pressure to reduce the cost of a patented medicine (Loff and Heywood 2002: 626). Developed countries and their pharmaceutical companies remain the largest financial beneficiaries from this international trade, *even after including the impact of the generic industry* (von Braun and Pugatch 2005: 602). In addition, even if we accept Resnik's figures pertaining to expenditure on R&D by the pharmaceutical industry, we should note that the burden is reduced by a combination of tax breaks and the substantial R&D support financed by the US federal government and national laboratories under the National Institutes of Health (NIH). This raises doubts about 'how much investment pharmaceutical companies actually provide in R&D and thus, to what extent a monopoly right in the form of a patent is justified' (von Braun and Pugatch 2005: 603).

Regardless of the minimal impact that generics may have on the profits of pharmaceutical companies, the rate of generic copying has intensified with Brazil and India (in particular) developing highly profitable pharmaceutical industries of their own (Subramanian 2004). In the case of most low- and middle-income countries, there were no regulations pertaining to pharmaceutical patents because there was no domestic pharmaceutical industry (Kumaranayake and Lake 2002: 91). It is worth noting that the TRIPS agreement allowed two exceptions: compulsory licensing (CL) and parallel importing (PI). Compulsory licensing allowed the manufacture of generic drugs without the agreement of the patent holder if a judicial or administrative body found this to be essential on the grounds of public interest (Kumaranayake and Lake 2002: 86). However, compensation to the patent holder was still expected. Parallel importing allowed for branded drugs to be purchased and imported from a third party in another country, enabling consumers to purchase an imported drug, provided it is sold at a lower price than in the drug's home country. Given this, the real impact of TRIPS was not the strict conditions under which TRIPS could permit generic production, but that TRIPS made it prohibitively expensive for a developing country to advance its own pharmaceutical industry, because of the cost associated with the licensing system (Shadlen 2007: 566–567).

Moreover, despite the allowances permitted by compulsory licensing and parallel importing, activists argue that the TRIPS system was unfairly balanced in favour of pharmaceutical companies. First, the right to produce under a licence could be delayed by patent holders beginning lengthy legal disputes to ensure that compulsory licensing exceptions were not allowed, halting generic production (Shadlen 2007). In addition, there was debate between international organizations, states and pharmaceutical companies about when a disease triggered 'public interest' and thereby opened the door to the compulsory licensing exception (WHO-WTO 2002: 234–235). For example, high-quality generic antiretroviral drugs are vital for more than half of those receiving treatment for HIV in the developing world, and most were produced after the 1994 TRIPS agreement. Therefore the approval of brand-name pharmaceutical companies is required for their generic production (Shadlen 2007: 564). Unsurprisingly, companies have been reluctant to give their consent, arguing that there is no public interest that outweighs their concerns about these drugs becoming generic. They also maintain that many of those countries seeking to produce generic versions lack the necessary technological capacity, that the cost of R&D for drug development would never be recouped which would mean no future equivalent of antiretrovirals, and finally that access to inexpensive drugs in poorly managed health care situations could lead to inaccurate dosage and increase the risk of drug resistance (Resnik 2001; Lippert 2002; Kaufmann 2006). The argument that inadequate public health sectors could increase the risk of inaccurate dosage is most apparent in debates about funding antiretroviral access in Africa. For example, in 2001 USAID administrator Andrew Natsios argued that 'sending antiretrovirals to African countries would be ineffective due to their lack of trained doctors, limited infrastructure, and the inability of Africans to follow a complicated treatment regimen because of their insufficient knowledge of clocks' (Dietrich 2007: 279).

Second, even when a state with a low-cost generic drug scheme was willing to sell to a third-party state, they were increasingly reluctant to do so after TRIPS, due to threats of drug price increases from pharmaceutical companies and political pressure from the United States (Thomas 2003: 182). Third, TRIPS provisions did not prevent sick individuals in low-income countries having to spend between 50% and 90% of their household income to afford essential drug treatment (Leach et al. 2005: 25–27). Finally, TRIPS provided no incentive for resolving the problem that tropical and preventable diseases account for approximately 90% of deaths each year, while only 10% of R&D expenditure was dedicated to new therapies for these diseases (Pogge 2005: 190).

The NGO movement led by MSF and governments in Brazil, South Africa and India campaigned against the 'effects of the WTO TRIPS agreement and its implementation at a national level' (Loff and Heywood 2002: 627; Ford 2004: 139). Campaigners positioned their call for access to medicine on health equity and human rights grounds:

> [T]he basic ability to deliver medical assistance in developing countries was being blocked by the global rules surrounding pharmaceutical drug production. On the one hand, the patent system was making drugs unaffordable for many people throughout the developing world and, on the other hand, it was doing little, if anything, to promote research and development of drugs for diseases that only affect the poor. (Ford 2004: 138–139)

This position was, of course, in direct opposition to the utilitarian perspectives of advocates of TRIPS. They countered that TRIPS should not be equated with access to drugs issues. For example, Attaran and Granville argue that 306 out of the 325 products listed on WHO's Essential Drug List no longer have patent protection (2004: 176). Instead, they argued, the main factor inhibiting the poor from gaining access to essential medicines was the absence of well-managed national public health sectors (Attaran and Granville 2004: 177). Furthermore, they maintained that devaluing patents could be 'counterproductive' – while the health equity proponents advocated a 'one size fits all' strategy, utilitarians argue that a careful consideration of which drugs may require patent protection to ensure future investment in R&D would be more appropriate (Attaran and Granville 2004: 179; Subramanian 2004: 24).

Before the Doha WTO Ministerial Round in November 2001, there was a renewed push by NGOs and generic producing countries including Brazil, South Africa and India (Loff and Heywood 2002: 627). This was largely the result of a South African litigation case resolved in the same year after forty multinational pharmaceutical companies and the South African Pharmaceutical Manufacturers Association attempted to block the South African government from introducing the Medicines Amendment Act (1997), which was to allow parallel imports, compulsory licensing and generic substitutions for antiretrovirals in particular, and medicines in general (Kongolo 2001: 609). The United States threatened South Africa with sanctions and the country was placed on the US Trade Representatives 'Trade Watch List' unless it repealed the Act or ensured the 'interests' of the American pharmaceutical industry (ibid.). The African Group of developing countries supported South Africa's fight against the pharmaceutical industry's attempt to block the Act, which itself came only after the Treatment Action Campaign had succeeded in a protracted struggle to persuade the South African government to take antiretroviral therapy seriously and as a public health measure (Ford 2004: 141). United States and European support for the pharmaceutical companies' action was challenged by a civil action trial in March 2001 (Ford 2004: 141). The level of outrage – within South Africa and across the continent – prompted the companies to drop the case and settle out of court (Kongolo 2001).[4] The concern for those campaigning against TRIPS was that this was only the tip of the iceberg. The TRIPS agreement had actually led to some states, including Bangladesh and Ghana, implementing even harsher regulations in order to retain the political favour of the United States and maintain important trade agreements (Thomas 2003; Harvey 2004; Shadlen 2007). Nor was the agreement clear about what should happen when microbial resistance to drugs on the WHO Essential Drug List occurred. Would arguments about costly technological equipment, R&D and patents prevent essential new drugs being made available to the world's poor (Ford 2004; Shadlen 2007)?

Under intense pressure, the Doha WTO Ministerial Round in 2001 attempted to clarify the 1994 TRIPS agreement with specific reference to the parallel importing and compulsory licensing articles and the measures states were allowed to take in order to protect public health. The Doha Ministerial Declaration on the TRIPS Agreement and Public Health stated that:

(b) Each member has the right to grant compulsory licenses and the freedom to determine the grounds upon which such licenses are granted.

(c) Each member has the right to determine what constitutes a national emergency or other circumstances of extreme urgency, it is being understood that public health crises, including those relating to HIV/AIDS, tuberculosis, malaria and other epidemics, can represent a national emergency or other circumstances of extreme urgency. (WTO 2001)

The Doha Declaration extended the obligation of member states to enforce patent protection from 2006 to 2016 for least developed countries. In cases where countries did not have manufacturing capacity to produce their own supply of drugs (which is the case for the majority of low-income countries in sub-Saharan Africa and some parts of Asia), alternative measures were to be identified. These states needed to be able to import generic versions, but 'importing a good presupposes someone else exporting that good, and TRIPS requires [Article 31.f] that goods produced in one country under a compulsory license be "predominantly" for domestic use' (Shadlen 2007: 567). Shadlen (2007: 568) notes that a group of developing countries had proposed that Article 30 of the TRIPS agreement be simplified to make 'foreign public health emergencies one such condition' where actors can 'use patented knowledge without obtaining any permissions from the state of the owner of the exclusive rights'. A drug company could, for example, produce a generic drug in one country and then supply it to a country that was experiencing a public health crisis (but without capacity to produce the drug locally) (Shadlen 2007: 568). However, strong pharmaceutical industry pressure prompted the United States, European Union and Switzerland to reject this proposal at the Doha Round.

It was not until 2003 that a solution to this particular problem – of countries being unable to produce generic drugs for public health emergencies – was found (Fleck 2003: 517; Hestermeyer 2007: 2). The 30 August 2003 agreement, reached after US objections to the Doha Declaration, involved a waiver of Article 31f (goods produced in one country under a compulsory licence are to be predominantly for domestic use) (Fleck 2003: 517; Curci and Vittori 2004: 746). Instead of the WTO members' original obligation to not produce for export, compulsory licences could now be granted to produce and export pharmaceutical products to 'eligible importing Members for *public health problems*' (emphasis added, Hestermeyer 2007: 2).

However, importing under this scheme required that all actors involved adhere to a number of conditions. First, the United States insisted that the Chair of the WTO Council attach a list of developing and developed countries that pledged not to use the system (Curci and Vittori 2004: 246; Shadlen 2007: 569). Importing countries were to ensure that they have a voluntary licence in place from the patent owner and if this is not available they could then seek a compulsory licence, and part of the licence determination requires the importing country to assess its own domestic generic industry capacity (to avoid waiver of Article 31f if the country is in fact able to produce the drug). If the country goes ahead with a compulsory licence request, it must then notify WTO of its decision, the quantity of the product it will seek and list the potential exporting country it plans to approach (Curci and Vittori 2004; 747). The exporting country must then issue its own licence limited to the quantity of drug necessary for the importing member country, with special packaging to identify that the drug has been sold under these conditions (to avoid attempts at parallel importing). The beneficiary must also post on a website the quantities received and distinguishing features of the product, before shipment (Hestermeyer 2007). Product registration is also required, and the WTO Council is empowered to conduct yearly reviews to ensure that all parties follow procedures and that there is no re-importing of the product (which would undermine the purpose of making the drugs available for a public health emergency) (Curci and Vittori 2004: 748).

The 2003 agreement was passed as a permanent mechanism in December 2005 by WTO members and it is now written into Article 31 of TRIPS and attached as an Annex to the agreement. The agreement of two-thirds of the WTO membership is required for the agreement to take effect – but as of 1 December 2007 only twelve of 151 WTO member states had accepted the amendment (Hestermeyer 2007: 2). Canada and Norway were the first and second countries to agree to the Article 31f waiver, followed by China, the European Union, South Korea and India in 2005. Each country has emphasized different requirements for drugs eligible for export and on whose behalf a petition for a licence can be made (Shadlen 2007: 569). MSF has criticized the rule, but was the first to test it in seeking access to three HIV/AIDS drugs. A Canadian company, Apotex, agreed in 2004 to produce the fixed dose combination of drugs that are patent owned by Glaxo Group, Wellcome Foundation, Shire Biochem, Boehringer Ingeheim and Dr Karl Thomae GmbH (Hestermeyer 2007: 2). However, Health Canada did not agree to license this new drug combination for MSF, to be produced by Apotex – first, because Apotex was having difficulty negotiating voluntary licences from patent holders, and second, because no developing country wanted to be named in the licence for fear of retribution and criticism (as happened with Thailand and Brazil when attempting similar deals) (Hestermeyer 2007: 2).[5] Rwanda eventually agreed to import the drug in May 2007 and notified the WTO Council of its intention. The Council circulated Rwanda's request in July and in September Apotex filed for a two-year compulsory licence to supply Rwanda with a specified quantity of drugs. In October 2007, Canada notified the WTO Council of the licence. As Hestermeyer argues, this process was clearly 'too cumbersome to work effectively' (2007: 3).

There is a cost to companies in having to wait for licence provisions (Shadlen 2007: 569). Shadlen argues that while the public momentum for making antiretroviral treatment available has worked to some extent in recent years, there is no guarantee that this will always work under the 2003 Agreement conditions. Aside from the most basic concerns about whether or not it will work if microbial resistance becomes an issue before the drug can reach the importing country, there are economic and political problems. There are very few firms involved with handling the Article 31f exemption. Changing this requires 'actors capable of securing public action for scaling up global treatment (i.e. the ability to demand compulsory licenses for export to poor people in poor countries) [with] few incentives to act, while actors needing action (i.e. people with HIV/AIDS in developing countries) may lack the necessary political resources' to demand such action (Shadlen 2007: 571). Moreover, activists (such as MSF and South Africa's Treatment Action Campaign) need to ensure that governments and private firms are willing to compete in a competitive market for 'politically risky and economically costly measures for poor people in other countries' (Shadlen 2007: 572), a difficult task to say the least. Finally, generic firms must operate in states that have not enacted patent acts that go beyond the requirements of WTO TRIPS and are willing to export according to the Article 31f waiver. However, the majority of developing states that are WTO members have already implemented TRIPS obligations – with patents on all pharmaceutical products – in spite of not needing to do so until 2016 (Forman 2007: 342; Shadlen 2007: 577).

In India, for example, there has already been a distinct change in its generic production of certain drugs due to the introduction of the Patent Act in 2005 and its increased bilateral dealings with multinational pharmaceutical companies (Sampath 2006). India's leading pharmaceutical companies are moving away from low-cost generics towards specialty generics that are designed primarily for the high-cost developed state drug market (Shadlen 2007: 574). As Forman argues, even if countries were willing to miss out on the benefits of bilateral trade agreements and endure trade sanctions by Western countries promoting the interests of their pharmaceutical industry, in the post-2016 environment, the twenty-year drug patents will make the WHO Essential Medicines List almost redundant (2007: 340–242).

In response to some of these problems, a study conducted on behalf of the UN Millennium Project Task Force on HIV/AIDS, Malaria, TB and Access to Essential Medicines presented a summary of recommendations that spoke to both health equity and utilitarian concerns (Leach et al. 2005). The Task Force argued that, while an effective health care system is essential for the purchase and distribution of drugs, the overwhelming factor limiting access to drugs is a lack of 'therapeutic innovation' (2005: 107). Essentially, states and international organizations such as WHO need to provide 'alternative international models to *the current patent-based system for priority setting and financing health R&D*' (Leach et al. 2005: 107). Medicines should be affordable and the best way to ensure this, the report argued, is to progressively increase public sector budgets (which will require government and donor government support) to reduce the costs to end users for essential medicines, and promote a transparent pharmaceutical financing mechanism that allows for the negotiation of pharmaceutical pricing based on a 'concept of equity' (Leach et al. 2005: 112–115).[6]

On the one hand, this working paper advocated improvement to public health sectors in the areas of the provision of health care workers, transparent and equitable funding mechanisms, and medicine registration systems to monitor use of pharmaceuticals, which is in keeping with the utilitarian concerns of those focusing on the efficiency of existing resources (Resnik 2001; Lippert 2002; Attaran and Granville 2004; Djolov 2004; Freeman 2006). On the other hand, the paper addressed the fact that the provision of public health in low-income countries does not exist in a vacuum, as the inability to fund public health is closely linked to the inequities inherent in the global political economy. The report noted that causes of unequal drug access range from WHO's inability to project a strong R&D model that can generate investment in 'neglected diseases', through to pharmaceutical companies being able to lobby their host government to enforce bilateral programmes that restrict 'best price' procurement and development (Leach et al. 2005: 107, 115). The study called for a pharmaceutical system based on the 'concept of equity', a strong nod to the health equity advocates who argue that, even if TRIPS is fair (and there are many questions about this), the political and economic factors surrounding its implementation are not (Thomas 2003; Lush 2004; von Braun and Pugatch 2005; Forman 2007; Shadlen 2007).

Unsurprisingly, this working paper was strongly criticized by the pharmaceutical industry. In fact, at the end of the report (Leach et al. 2005: app. 2) is a 'statement of dissent' by the representatives of the research-based pharmaceutical industry who were involved in the Working Group. They argued that the working paper's link between patent protection and poor access to medicine did not reflect the main source of the problem and was not a fair reflection of the pharmaceutical industry's pricing practices. Instead, they argued, there was an 'inaccurate and subjective link forged between rights, "monopoly" pricing, and global inequities in access to medicines' (2005: 138). A year later, the US Department of State published a document, *Focus on Intellectual Property Rights*, which supported this view, arguing that 'violating or bypassing patent protections is a short-term solution that threatens long-term health of the world's citizens by removing the incentives and discouraging the innovation we need' (Kaufmann 2006: 81).

Therefore, the TRIPS agreement and the political debates that followed it are far from solving the problem of access to essential medicines (Cullet 2003; Attaran and Granville 2004; Santoro 2005; Cohen et al. 2006). As Barry and Raworth argue:

> [D]ebate concerning rules governing intellectual property may be one example of a wider phenomenon: we all focus intensely on the tip of the institutional iceberg because *only that* is above water. If, however, participants on both sides of debates concerning global problems fail to consider the unfairness of deeper and older aspects of international order . . . their allocations of remedial responsibility for global problems may well be dangerously distorted. (2002: 70)

While Attaran and Granville (2004) are correct to argue that, even if drugs could be provided at low or no cost to the world's poorest, these populations would still lack access to affordable health care, we should acknowledge that low-cost drugs would make a great difference to many in the developing world who spend 50–90% of their wages on drugs. Imagine if this income was made available for investment in schooling, sanitation and food. To be sure, antiretroviral drug resistance is potentially a huge problem, but the long-lasting effects of HIV-infected populations contracting increasingly drug-resistant TB or hepatitis C because they are not receiving affordable antiretroviral treatment poses a huge problem too. Expenditure on R&D is vital to ensure that treatment is available in the first place but, as shown above, patents do not have a zero-sum relationship to R&D. as is often suggested. The majority of innovative pharmaceutical discoveries have been achieved through government-sponsored research. The disparity that 90% of drug and disease R&D is focused on diseases affecting only 20% of the world's population has not improved because of TRIPS. Utilitarians are right to argue that removing TRIPS will not solve the problems faced by fractured health care systems in the developing world, but health equity advocates are also right to argue that TRIPS has done nothing to reduce this inequity and, worse, has added additional burdens onto the world's most vulnerable and those who seek to care for them.

Offshore clinical trials

The capacity of the pharmaceutical industry to shape an individual's health is immense, whether it is through financing the creation of an essential drug or control of production and distribution of that drug. Perhaps the most direct influence, however, is through the link between clinical drug trials and primary health care checks – shaping the level and type of care that individuals can access in low income countries. Offshore clinical trials now account for over 40% of the approximately 50,000 studies taking place in any given year, worldwide. No precise data is available on the spread of drug testing and types of drug between regions, because many national drug associations do not have precise data on the number of experiments involving new drug trials (Petryna 2007: 21). This is the result, Dickersin and Rennie argue, of 'industry resistance, the lack of funding appropriation for a serious and sustained effort [to regulate], lack of a mechanism for enforcement policies, and lack of awareness of the importance of the problem' (2003: 516). It is estimated that between 1990 and 1999 there has been a 16-fold increase in offshore clinical testing (Reed et al. 2007: 492). Meanwhile the number of private contract research organizations (CROs) conducting testing has also increased, with pharmaceutical companies reducing the proportion of tests conducted by universities from 80% in 1990 to only 35% in 2005 (Fisher 2006: 678).

Utilitarians point to the dearth of R&D dedicated to tropical diseases and argue that conducting trials among the populations most affected is an excellent way of ensuring quality control for the drug and patients, as it maintains a link between pharmaceutical research and the developing world (Crooks 2005; Mytelka 2006; Wechsler 2006). On the other hand, those advocating the health equity perspective question whether the attachments of 'strings' to the provision of health care is a form of coercion, particularly in low-income countries where ill patients may simply agree to be participants in new drug trials in return for receiving basic medical care (Annas and Grodin 1999; Angell 2004; Luna 2006). Worse still, sometimes patients may not even know that they are taking part in a drug trial (Shah 2006: 87; Petryna 2007: 28, 30). Thus, some complain that 'African patients are being used as guinea pigs for untested Western medicines, a scientific exploitation that one rarely hears about' (Horton 2003: 169).

There are a number of reasons why Western-owned pharmaceutical companies are moving their clinical trials offshore to low-income countries. Since 1987, the US Food and Drug Administration (FDA) has allowed new drug applications based on data exclusively gathered from overseas trials (Shah 2006: 7). While drug trials have been contracted out since the 1970s (Petryna 2007: 25), the increased market value of drug companies and the economic benefits of patenting new drugs and marketing them as the 'cure all' for a particular disease led to a proliferation of CROs stating that they could reduce the drug testing and approval time-frame from ten years to four (Petryna 2007: 26). In addition, the rise in public relations disasters for brand-name drug companies due to past testing practices (see below) also made CROs an attractive proposition. Tests could still be conducted – but by a contract organization – allowing the drug company to distance itself from any bad publicity. This solved a huge problem facing drug companies and reduced the time needed for testing and approval by finding people willing to volunteer for particular clinical tests.

Negative reactions to the testing of disabled and mentally ill patients between the 1950s and 1980s, and the 1980 ban on testing prisoners in the United States (before this ban, up to 90% of drugs licensed in the United States had been tested on prison populations), meant that there were too few human volunteers in developed countries when the number of drugs needing testing was expanding (Shah 2006: 6–8; Petryna 2007: 32).[7] Within this context, pharmaceutical companies and CROs looked to the developing world for volunteers, people who were not aware of this prob-lematic past and who were willing to trust people in white coats (Petryna 2007). There was also an economic incentive for exporting drug trials to low-income countries where 'reimbursement for health care services may be small relative to payments for participation in clinical research' (Reed et al. 2007: 492). As a result, the combination of an increasingly competi-tive pharmaceutical industry, CROs willing to run the trials offshore, a reduced number of 'first world' volunteers and the relatively low cost of testing patients in the developing world all contributed to the rapid rise of offshore clinical trials.

Offshore clinical testing has produced mixed results thus far. Its pro-ponents argue that poor populations gain access to better regular health care through participating in trials. However, this increased access is marginal at best and comes at a significant cost. The power of the phar-maceutical industry is 'accentuated in developing countries where the government and health department has limited resources and negotiating power' to regulate behaviour of these companies (Weston 1999: 5). In the international sphere, pharmaceutical companies are often able to exert more influence collectively than developing countries. Thus, for instance, at a joint WTO-WHO meeting on the pricing of essential medicines, of the eighty participants there were fewer than ten representatives from developing countries, but sixteen pharmaceutical industry representatives.

This imbalance was also evident at the WTO Doha meeting that same year (Lush 2002: 236).

Within the countries where offshore clinical trials are taking place, there is an inadequate number of health care clinics and basic medical equipment is often lacking. As a result, public health ministries may be encouraged to trade their responsibility to provide health care to pharmaceutical companies that are willing to provide such care in return for participation in clinical trials (Angell 2004). For example, Malawi spends a higher proportion of its GDP on public health (about 2.5–3% more) than does India – a state with the highest percentage GDP increase this decade (Attaran and Granville 2004: 185; Conroy et al. 2004: 53). Despite this increased investment in health, Malawi's investment only amounts to $5–6 per person each year on health. However, the government wanted to put in place an Essential Healthcare Package to stem the spread of HIV, TB and malarial infections in its population; this package was estimated to cost $22 per person – well above Malawi's health expenditure (Conroy et al. 2004: 53). What option does a government have in such a situation but to accept public–private partnerships with pharmaceutical companies, or to engage in deals with CROs wanting to test new therapies in return for health investment (Buse and Walt 2002; Heaton 2004)?

Another issue linked to testing practice is the 'placebo trial'. Since the 1970s, there has been an emphasis on placebo controls, as they are seen as being rather effective in measuring the efficacy of active treatments. Indeed, the US FDA argues that it prefers placebo-controlled trials (Shah 2006: 32). However, placebo trials are morally problematic when the people being tested do not know that a placebo treatment involves no actual therapy, and that the placebo may be delivered in place of a therapy that works in order to test a new drug. While the second sort of trial is unethical and forbidden in Article 29 in the 2002 Declaration of Helsinki, *Ethical Principles for Medical Research Involving Human Subjects* (www.wma.net/e/policy/b3.html), prior to the Declaration such trials did occur. For instance, in 1992, a trial on HIV-infected pregnant women was conducted to determine antiretroviral effectiveness in preventing mother-to-child HIV transmission. Professor Jay Brooks Jackson designed a study to compare two different types of antiretroviral treatment with a third group that had no treatment at all (Shah 2006: 87). When asked about this Jackson replied that 'the current standard of care [in Uganda] involves no antiretroviral therapy . . . ethically . . . this study will not deny women access to a proven therapy to which they would otherwise have access' (Shah 2006: 87). The argument used in this case, and similar cases where people have been used for placebo effect trials, is that if they were not receiving a treatment prior to the trial then they are technically not being denied access to treatment (Angell 1997; Lurie and Wolfe 1997; de Zulueta 2001).

Those involved in a placebo trial may still believe that they are contributing to a new therapy, or that they are taking part in the trial for alternative benefits such as health care checks, payment (if provided) or meals (if provided) (Fisher 2006: 691; Shah 2006: 149–151). Brody (2002: 202) argues that as long as participants have been informed in a 'culturally sensitive fashion' and they demonstrate understanding of the placebo effect, 'there seems to be little reason to be concerned about coercion simply because a good opportunity is being offered to those individuals with few opportunities'. However, there are important conflicts of interest between care and experimentation when hospitals and health care clinics are conducting trials on behalf of the pharmaceutical industry (Fisher 2006; Shah 2006: 173). First, such trials require that one group of people believe they are receiving treatment when they are not. Second, CROs often seek access to participants in low-income countries through medical facilities, and people will agree to trials more readily in hospital settings in the belief that they will receive some form of health therapy (Petryna 2007). Therefore, in countries where health care standards are already poor, ill people may subject themselves to a drug trial in the hope of receiving care *and treatment*. As a result, in regions such as Africa where ethical standards committees are rare, there is little oversight to ensure that participants are being treated according to the Declaration of Helsinki principles for ethical research (Horton 2003: 169).

Proponents argue that clinical trials and the provision of health care may provide minimal care in a context where there are few other options (Resnik 1998; Brody 2002). In the Ugandan example, while a third of the women in the trial were not receiving any treatment to prevent HIV transmission to their child, there was no guarantee when the trial commenced that the two HIV therapies would make a difference (though it should be mentioned that one soon did). Is it enough that these women and their children received regular medical check-ups that they might not have received otherwise? How far should those testing a drug go to ensure that the potential participants are aware that they may not receive any medical benefit from participating in a trial? These concerns revolve around the question of free will. Drug trials rely on volunteers giving their consent with full knowledge of what they are consenting to (Annas and Grodin 1999; Luna 2006). How can we ever know whether participants in Uganda or Bangalore participate in a drug trial because they would freely choose to do so regardless, or because they believe that their participation will give them care that they would not otherwise have access to? The concern is that these participants' economic and health needs are being exploited for the benefit of pharmaceutical companies, and that the reason for increased drug trials in low- and middle-income countries is because in these countries people are to be found who are desperate to avoid the high costs of health care for their medical conditions. As a result, the benefits to the participants are incidental.[8] Moreover, the lack of continued care makes these populations vulnerable to toxicity reactions (Reed et al. 2007: 498). However, CROs rarely attempt to improve the long-term health of participants and therefore individuals are being used for a short term (economic) benefit in a manner that exploits their physical, economic and political vulnerability.

The 2002 Declaration of Helsinki on medical research ethics has come under criticism for not containing follow-through mechanisms so that local ethics committees are able to freely verify that drug testing occurred with no 'strings attached' and that individual consent was given freely and in full knowledge of the implications (Petryna and Kleinman 2006). Ironically, others worry that the real victim in all of this could be the 'naïve US company that steps into such a situation [offshore testing]' who 'may be easily victimized by unscrupulous suppliers or individuals' and only wanted to 'take advantage of the unused capacity in a foreign country' (Kuwahara 2007: 30). Arguably if those countries that are host to the majority of pharmaceutical companies were to 'incentivize' pharmaceutical interest in the diseases of the developing world, it would contribute to improving overall health levels in these countries and resolve some concerns about who really benefits from offshore clinical testing (Selgelid and Sepers 2006). In contrast, many argue that the only attraction developing countries pose to pharmaceutical companies is the large numbers of 'new test subjects' that are 'treatment-naïve' (Shah 2006: 105). Patients who do not have access to medication, are ill and desperate for medical attention make excellent test subjects, cynics might argue. Indeed, some point out the irony that the majority of new drugs coming out today have been tested on populations that cannot afford them, and the pharmaceutical industry is still able to maintain support for its argument that patents are justified in such conditions (MacDonald 2007; Petryna 2007).

Where we go from here is back to the questions posed by the debate about essential medicines. IPEH now has a number of private actors that can assist 'public' health systems, and a number of public actors that have little positive impact on their citizens' health. Offshore clinical trials reflects this dilemma most starkly – CROs can provide health care (albeit temporarily) and public health systems can be relieved of health costs by allowing such trials to take place. The key problem with offshore clinical trials is ascertaining whether consent is informed and freely given and determining who ultimately benefits most from testing drugs in low-income countries. If big pharmaceutical companies are able to test their drugs in a short timeframe, sick people are able to access the drugs sooner or access medical care not otherwise available to them, and the public health system saves or perhaps makes some money, then haven't the greatest number benefited? The problem, health equity proponents argue, is the lack of safeguards for when things go wrong and the lack of commitment to long-term health. There is no health care structure that sick people in poor countries can fall back on when a trial goes wrong, no protection for people participating in a placebo trial, and the free medical clinic is closed after the trial ends. On balance, it is fairly clear that the negative consequences of offshore clinical testing outweigh the possible good. To start with, we need to be careful when talking about 'participants' in such situations where poverty is exploited to coerce consent. Moreover, many of the people tested may never be able to afford the drugs for which they offered their bodies for trials. Finally, ethical standards cannot be enforced in situations where public health ministries have difficulty providing primary health care needs. In sum, what makes offshore clinical trials attractive to stakeholders – both states and private actors – is precisely what makes them dangerous. Without clear safeguards, the process is left open to abuse and the greater risk is that it damages rather than improves people's health.

Vaccination projects

One of the great advances of the twentieth century was the eradication of smallpox. WHO's vertical programme to eradicate smallpox by mass vaccination meant that the last naturally occurring outbreak was in Somalia in 1977, and by 1979 WHO was able to declare the disease officially eradicated (Harrison 2004: 183; Bonita et al. 2007: 269). The eradication of smallpox was a rare achievement for the WHO. The Cold War rivalry between the United States and the USSR was a key conduit for smallpox eradication, with competition leading to the United States seeking to provide expert assistance to the vaccination programme and the Soviet Union providing most of the vaccine (Harrison 2004: 184; Allen 2007: 12). Today, we see a similar zeal to end preventable disease through vaccine, but by different actors. In this section, I examine the growth of private actors in the allocation of expenditure on health projects for the world's poor. Vaccinations putatively meet the requirements of both utilitarian and health equity proponents, and could even be seen as resolving the tension between the statist and globalist perspectives. Vaccinations are a low-cost equitable treatment made available to everyone in danger of dying from preventable disease and provide long-term protection from disease. However, similar to the concerns expressed in relation to access to medicines and offshore clinical trials, focusing on the delivery of vaccines by external actors potentially neglects the broader health inequity and public health incapacities that have caused the low vaccination rate in the first place.

The Gates Foundation has been instrumental in leading a resurgent vaccination drive against diseases that strike the poorest and most vulnerable. Leading vaccination funding efforts since 1999 (Allen 2007: 435) in the areas of malaria, TB, HIV/AIDS, measles and diarrhoeal disease, the Gates Foundation's investment has totalled $8 billion (*Economist* 2008). Since leading the vaccination drive through the Global Alliance for Vaccine and Immunization (GAVI) in 1999 (see chapter 2), the Gates Foundation has invested in the top ten pharmaceutical companies and in technology transfer agreements with developing states that can utilize the technology for further health sector know-how (Allen 2007: 437; Carlin 2008: 27–29; *Economist* 2008). While contention has increased about the number of children actually being vaccinated against the common diseases that plague childhood, such as measles, diphtheria, pertussis, rubella, polio and tetanus (Murray et al. 2007), investment in vaccine research has continued at a breakneck pace thanks largely to the Gates Foundation's ambition to provide technology-based solutions to diseases such as malaria, where all other proposed 'magic bullets' have failed (Carlin 2008: 27). A recent example is the Gates Foundation's announcement of progress in the Advanced Market Commitment (AMC) project that, in conjunction with Canada, Italy, Norway, Russia and the United Kingdom, will pay for a vaccine to protect children against pneumonia and meningitis (Anderson 2008b: 43). The project has been in development since 2005 and has recently secured the $1.5 billion required to launch. There are few cheap vaccines available to combat both diseases in Africa and Asia, and the AMC will accelerate the development of an affordable vaccine to be distributed in poor countries at a subsidized price.

But what are the limitations of relying on vaccination programmes for the 'magic bullet'? Some question whether a malarial vaccine, for example, is the 'magic bullet' – arguing that old-fashioned programmes that seek to improve public health systems may in fact be more effective for preventing malaria in the long run (Kochi in McNeil 2008). Alternative anti-malaria strategies are seen to be particularly important due to the resistance of malarial mosquitoes to eradication and vaccination efforts in the past (Birn 2005). Treated bed nets, spraying the walls of homes with insecticides and testing ancient herbal remedies have also led to gains in some regions – up to 77% reduction rates in Zambia and Tanzania (Anderson

2008a). Scepticism towards vaccination as the primary prevention strategy for illnesses is also based on cultural concerns about vaccine delivery. In 2002 the mainly Muslim state of Kono in Nigeria boycotted a national polio immunization day in the belief that the vaccine was contaminated with hormones that would create infertility and even carried the AIDS virus. One of the local opponents, a Kano physician and president of Nigeria's Supreme Council for Sharia Law, argued that the United States was promoting the vaccine with the purpose of genocide (Allen 2007: 440). This occurred in a country where only 25% of the children were vaccinated in 2002 compared to 50% coverage ten years earlier (Roberts 2006: 5). While this reaction in Kono might bring despair to those wanting to save children from a crippling disease, it exemplifies the deeper problems with trying to ensure that communities *own* their health care programmes, which is necessary if they are to be sustainable in the long term.

Former US CDC director, William Foege, argues that 'immunization is a foundation stone for all modern public health . . . And if you can't run a vaccine program it's not likely you can do other things' (Foege in Allen 2007: 44). Vaccination programmes may therefore be blocked by a variety of factors and a programme may not be able to achieve the coverage originally expected. An inadequate number of health care workers to distribute the vaccine, community resistance, and the waxing and waning of donor interest all contribute to the premature end of vaccination projects. To what extent, then, should the extent of vaccination programmes be an indicator of effective public health care interventions?

A 2006 study on the progress of GAVI, for instance, showed that while there had been an increase in diphtheria, tetanus and pertussis (DTP3) vaccinations in countries where coverage was below 50% (between 1995 and 2004), there were difficulties in increasing coverage in countries where DTP3 coverage was 65% (Lu et al. 2006). The cause of this appeared to be a correlation between the per capita cost of the vaccination and the level of coverage: in countries where there was poor vaccination coverage the GAVI funding increased coverage. In countries where coverage was above 65% but below 80%, GAVI funding seemed to have no effect. GAVI has argued that this means that funding needs to be concentrated on countries with low immunization rates, but these figures may also indicate that there are fundamental problems with health care coverage that affects the programme's ability to cross the 65% threshold and ensure long-term delivery and support. Sustaining vaccine coverage over the long term and expanding it beyond the initial vaccination drive requires strong public health systems. In 2005, GAVI's total funding was $760.5 million; of which only $124–125 million, or 16% of total GAVI funds, went to immunization support services (ISS) which included personnel, infrastructure and support for national health systems (Lu et al. 2006).

An additional problem to ensuring the development of basic health infrastructure in conjunction with vaccination programmes is the 'push' mechanisms for vaccine development (Lieu et al. 2005). Vaccines have historically only accounted for 1.5% of global pharmaceutical sales because their purchase price is very low compared to other drugs (Lieu et al. 2005). The push for a malaria vaccine by the Gates Foundation has meant a quadrupling of the foundation's funding for vaccine development to $1 billion since 2000 (Carlin 2008: 28). The importance of the Gates investment in vaccine development cannot be underestimated – it leads to companies such as GlaxoSmithKline agreeing to assist with the development, manufacture and testing of the vaccine (Carlin 2008). Investment incentives are vital for such companies, which need to be continually aware of the market benefits for such investment (Buckup 2008). As one of the Gates-funded researchers working on the malaria vaccine in Tanzania put it, '[t]hat is the reality in the capitalist world and it's no use screaming about it . . . Because the truth is that if we don't have Big Pharma, we don't have the products' (Carlin 2008: 29).

Thus, public–private partnerships in the area of vaccine production and delivery by private actors such as the Gates Foundation, Rotary International, pharmaceutical companies such as Merck and GlaxoSmithKline, and international organizations including UNICEF and WHO, has led to real momentum in the campaign to eradicate diphtheria, tetanus, pertussis, polio and measles. But will it produce long-term gains in health? The allegation remains that GAVI spends more money on developing new vaccines than on ensuring that existing ones are being delivered through a well-financed immunization support programme – which would build public health infrastructure and contribute to the training of local health care workers (Birn 2005). Lieu et al. (2005) also argue that it remains to be seen whether these new vaccines will remain affordable in the long term, and whether research into new vaccine development will continue to be a priority if donor interest and cost 'effectiveness' wane for a moment.

Most troubling, perhaps, is the prioritization of vaccination over support for strengthened health systems when the evidence suggests that both are required. Vaccination delivery programmes that focus on scientific and technical improvements are increasingly being seen as the solution. In part, I would argue, this is because it is easier to invest in vaccines than to engage in the long-term politics necessary to build public health systems and the vaccines are desperately needed in remote areas where there is no access to immediate health care (Anderson 2008a: 43). Because of the utility of vaccinations, developing states rarely refuse assistance for vaccine delivery programmes, there have even been ceasefires during conflicts to ensure immunization coverage in Sudan, Ethiopia, DRC and Angola.

However, getting the financial and policy support required to ensure a long-term gain from vaccinations is harder. It requires donor states to make a long-term commitment to health improvements at the local level, for recipient states to prioritize health care, for donor states to relieve debt and allow recipient states to invest in public health programmes, and for private partners such as the Gates Foundation and pharmaceutical companies to transfer their technological discoveries to local clinics and laboratories.

Here, we come full circle and see the other reason why investment beyond vaccination is difficult. A holistic approach to health care is more complex and multifaceted. The moment a child is vaccinated she will be protected for life from diseases such as measles and diphtheria; but she is not protected from filthy water, malnutrition and poor sanitation. As Shereen Usdin argues, mass immunization programmes are vital for making significant inroads in child survival, but they are narrow in focus and 'broader strategies to improve health get neglected, including the strengthening of the health system as a whole' (2007: 21). Investment in vaccination programmes is relatively low cost with immediate benefit to a population, as a utilitarian would argue. However, as health equity advocates are also right to argue, successful vaccination projects need to build on the short-term gains of vaccination programmes and secure long-term gains with health workers, clean water, and access to food, shelter and affordable medicines. It is important, therefore, that vaccination programmes be seen as part of a broader strategy to strengthen public health systems, not as a replacement for such a strategy. External actors, especially philanthropic organizations, have begun to play a crucial role in vaccination programmes precisely because this is one health intervention that has immediate demonstrable impact. However, sustainable health requires long-term investment, deep engagement and partnership with public health systems by both external actors and programme recipient states.

Health tourism

Malaysian Tourism Minister, Datuk Seri Tengku Adnan Tengku Mansor, launched a 'Malaysia health care' tourism website on 1 May 2007 in Dubai to promote Malaysia as the 'one stop destination for all your medical and tourism related needs' (Malaysia Ministry of Health 2007). Health tourism in countries such as India, Malaysia, Singapore and Thailand has grown thanks to the General Agreement on Trade in Services (GATS), which allows 'consumption abroad'. Consumption abroad refers to the 'movement of consumers/patients and students to foreign countries for treatment and education' (Ranson et al. 2002: 33). While utilitarians argue that GATS allows 'increased trade in health services [which] could open the sector to increased competition, bringing with it needed technology and management expertise, and for some countries, increased earnings' (Ranson et al. 2002: 32), those concerned with health equity maintain that 'there is little evidence on whether and how the additional incomes and resources from health tourism have been leveraged to improve national health systems' (Blouin 2007: 91). This section explores whether countries with the capacity to provide relatively standard health care to their citizens have a responsibility to do so, or whether the provision of health care should be considered a resource available to those who can afford it for the long-term benefit of the state's economic development.

Health tourism clearly puts pressure on public health systems and creates shortages of health care workers. However, health tourism is estimated to be worth $60 billion a year and growing at 20% each year. India alone will receive $2.2 billion into its economy by 2012 from medical tourists (MacReady 2007: 1849). Patients from the United States, in particular, are increasingly seeking health tourism 'packages' because medical procedures can be conducted far more cheaply in countries like India than in their home country, and patients can then recuperate in 'luxury Asian resorts' (MacReady 2007: 1850). For example, Anne Marie Moncure, managing director of Apollo Hospitals in New Delhi, is 'upbeat on the potential for medical tourism, pointing out that around 50 million Americans are uninsured, with even the insured having to pay substantial amounts for treatment' (Deshpande 2005: 1). Likewise, Australians seeking cosmetic procedures in particular are flocking to Malaysia and Thailand, and British patients who are tired of waiting on NHS lists are travelling to India and Thailand for medical procedures (Nambiar 2004: 2; Deshpande 2005: 1; Sen 2005: 1; MacReady 2007: 1850).

Furthermore, there is evidence that as health tourism competition has increased in Asia, there have been calls for more aggressive investment by the state in this niche market. In India, Naresh Trehan, a cardiologist for Escorts Heart Institute, is building a medical city in Gurgaon with 2,000 beds intended for the exclusive use of overseas patients. Dr Trehan argues that 'We [India] need to get our act together and deliver quality services consistently, get accreditation and have uniform prices' (Deshpande 2005: 1). Thailand is becoming one of the most popular destinations, with patients including the wealthy from Laos, Cambodia, Myanmar, Bangladesh, Sri Lanka and the Middle East. In response, health tourism advocates in India have expressed concern at Thailand's increased popularity, with health tourism agencies arguing that what distinguishes Thailand's medical care from India's is 'the service-orientation. Each private hospital has a dedicated international patients centre that looks more like five-star hotel lounges' (Sen 2005: 1). In response, India's market leaders insist that India needs to become more resort-like to secure the health tourism market.

Of course, it could be argued that such concerns miss the larger point. The real problem is that there is no way of determining the extent to which the additional income generated by health tourism has delivered direct benefit to the national health systems in these countries (Blouin 2007: 91). In India, diseases such as cholera and malaria are still rife among poor populations, and the risk is that health tourism turns attention to specialized hospitals that cater for foreign patients in preference to treating large numbers of India's poor (Blouin 2007: 90). India's health costs are primarily paid from private sources, mainly from household incomes, thus health expenses are directly linked to continued impoverishment among the rural poor (Blouin 2007: 92; Usdin 2007: 24). Therefore, while India's poor pay exorbitant costs for health care (comparative to their income), the Indian government invests in the health tourism sector. This could mean, Blouin (2007) argues, that health tourism may benefit the Indian economy by boosting health investments; but as yet there appears to be no direct benefit to the poor and those most reliant on the rapidly diminishing public health care system.

Furthermore, with the inevitably higher wages and prestige associated with working for private hospitals, there is also the increased potential for a shortage of public health workers. In Singapore, for example, 48% of doctors work in the public sector and admit 79% of all inpatients, in contrast to the private sector which has more physicians but four times fewer inpatients (Blouin 2007: 90). Health tourism also encourages the migration of health care workers to countries with higher wages. In Indonesia, which has an understaffed health care system, there is increased concern that the attraction of working in the high-wage private health industry in Malaysia and Singapore is further exacerbating domestic health worker shortages (Arunanondchai and Fink 2007: 62).

In Thailand, there has been no policy initiative to deal with the loss of health professionals in the public sector, resulting in a shortage of medical doctors in public hospitals, especially in rural areas. Malaysia is also suffering from shortages of medical personnel, which could start to affect the positive outcomes that it has made in primary health care over the last thirty years (Beaglehole and Bonita 2004: 244; Arunanondchai and Fink 2007: 63).

However, proponents claim that the burgeoning of a competitive private health care industry spurred on by health tourism can produce stronger local health care initiatives (Frenk et al. 2001). They refer to the increase of public and private hospitals in Kuala Lumpur, and the growth of

24-hour-seven-days-a-week clinics for local and foreign nationals in Jakarta (Frenk et al. 2001: 38). On balance, such initiatives are so small and infrequent that the growth of the private industry has led to a two-tier health system of health care, in which good treatment requires high out-of-pocket expenses for patients and, in these health tourism countries, very few local patients are able to access the excellent treatment provided in the private hospitals. There is also little evidence that the money generated by health tourism has increased investment in the public health sector in these countries.

While advocates of health tourism avoid addressing the consequences of a vastly unequal health care system, they do point out that visa-free travel for health visits and portable health insurance plans within the region improves the liberalization of health trade (Arunanondchai and Fink 2007: 64). The outward migration of health workers is acknowledged as a problem, but their solution is the creation of short-term visas that would require health care workers to return to their home country after receiving specialist medical training. Arunanondchai and Fink (2007: 66) actually argue that further regional integration will improve the health care market and deliver stronger regulation and health capacity. However, they do not address the problem of ensuring that health care service improvements will benefit all, not just wealthy local citizens and tourists.

Overall, health tourism benefits only a small section of the local population, and draws people and resources away from the public health sector. Health tourism contributes little to health improvement for the local population from a utilitarian or health equity perspective. Health workers are lost from an already overburdened public health system and there is no evidence that it provides any investment into public health in these countries. In short, it could be argued that health tourism reflects an area where developing states have the power to prevent wealthy actors from exploiting their health systems, or at least to ensure that the underprivileged benefit from such investment, but in most cases explored here these states are all too willing to simply compromise the health of their poor for gains to a privileged few.

Conclusion

In this chapter I have sought to highlight how IPEH understands health challenges from two different approaches. Health can be approached from a utilitarian perspective, where health resources are distributed according to principles of cost effectiveness and financial sustainability, or from a health equity perspective which insists that resources should be directed towards delivering on a basic right to health for all. In relation to access to medicines, offshore clinical trials, vaccination projects and health tourism, I have demonstrated that there are a proliferation of actors beyond the state, such as pharmaceutical companies, NGOs, private foundations and private health care providers. Reflecting the themes developed in chapter 2, this chapter has demonstrated that within the international political economy of health non-state actors can influence the health of individuals, and have a degree of influence that can sometimes rival that of states. As a result, and as evidenced in all of the four cases, low- and middle-income states in particular are struggling to come to terms with a range of new pressures and constraints. While the statist and globalist perspectives both encourage states to build the public health capacity required to respond to their citizens' health needs, the reality is that this capacity can be constrained by external economic forces beyond state control. In order to improve their health capacity, states sometimes take advantage of the opportunities presented by globalization, such as health tourism and offshore clinical trials. These avenues involve the state making a calculated choice to withdraw from their role in the delivery of health care. The result is that the tension is not resolved – the state may remain unable or unwilling to accommodate the needs of its citizens and global actors seek to either accommodate or exploit individual needs. But the need for both state and global actors to work together remains in each of the cases explored in this chapter. Until then, debate will remain squarely focused on the apparent competition between responding to the health needs of individuals and the health priorities of the state.

CONCLUSION

Why should International Relations (IR) seek to contribute an analytical perspective on health? Our answer largely depends on whether we believe that the current issues that we identify as important in world politics exist independent of any other factors that affect the daily lives of people around the world. If Richard Price (2008: 19–20) is right and IR's subject matter is determined merely by the fact that we have yet to fully appreciate the full range of interests and concerns that shape world politics, then we must begin to develop a more comprehensive understanding of our subject matter. When we consider the wider effects of persistent poor health in fragile societies or the massive indirect deaths caused by war, it is not hard to see that there is a degree of interdependence between public health concerns and global politics.

I argued in the introduction that IR needs to more closely examine the interdependence between health and politics and that this interdependence operates at the global level, the local level, at every level in between, and between the levels themselves. However, only rarely does IR treat health as an important dependent variable in its own right. For instance, the quality of health care available to a given population may be a contributing element to a situation of international concern, but it would rarely be considered as a key factor. Particular health issues tend only to generate global political interest when it is deemed to be important for the state's survival (Booth 1996: 337; Buzan et al. 1998a: 388–390). The dependent variable is the survival of the state rather the various conditions, parameters and elements concerning health at the local, international and global levels themselves (George and Bennett 2005: 79). The result is that IR has neglected an empirically rich area of relations between states and relations between states and non-state actors.

The public health issues that I have examined – health and human rights, the health needs of cross-border migrants and refugees, health and armed conflict, preventing the spread of infectious disease, and the international political economy of health – involve a broad range of actors both within and outside the state. In different ways, these actors constitute the ideational and material structures that determine the level of health care available at the local level. Critically, each of these issues has become global, not just international, because each involves the complex interplay of state and non-state actors – local, national, regional, international and global. In chapter 1, I identified two prominent perspectives on the global politics of health – statist and globalist. Then, in chapter 2, I mapped some of the key actors that operate within the global politics of health and frame global health governance. What became evident in these chapters is that, while both statist and globalist perspectives had their own strengths and limitations, together they helped illuminate some of the key tensions that inform the contemporary global politics of health. In the chapters that followed, I examined five issues, each of which provided evidence of these tensions in practice: the issue of health as a human right; the relationship between health and migration; war and health; the prevention and containment of infectious disease; and the international political economy of health. In each of these cases, I argued that a tension was apparent between the state's identity as the primary actor in protecting health and responding to individual needs, and the reality that the state was often unwilling or incapable of fulfilling this role. This in turn has created a role for a variety of external and non-state actors. However, the convergence of these actors has more often than not furthered the tension between the putative rights and needs of states, and the rights and needs of individuals. The result is a duality in international health policy that permeates the politics of human rights, refugee and migration practices, conflict management, international health law and the international economy of health.

In the case of human rights, this tension is specifically rooted in the idea that individuals have a right to health that can only be realized through the state. As we saw in the cases of HIV/AIDS and reproductive health, states will often seek to protect their own political interests or cultural practices rather than help realize the rights owed to vulnerable individuals. In the area of cross-border migration, we saw a similar prioritization of states' putative interests that came at the cost of protecting refugee and migrant populations and damaging the health of all. In the case of refugees, humanitarian actors sometimes try to compensate for the neglect of state actors by providing health services. Likewise, when host states associate migrants with health 'threats' they place these populations at greater health risk. Precisely the same logic was evident in debates about how best to respond to infectious diseases. This issue has become prominent in IR through the successful securitization of infectious disease, which means that powerful states see such diseases as potentially existential threats and therefore grant extra resources to them. The consequence has been that attention has been drawn away from the broader range of communicable diseases, which actually afflict more people. In the case of contemporary armed conflict, in addition to a number of pivotal questions relating, for instance, to how we count the dead, this duality was reflected in the withdrawal of the state from the provision of health care and the dilemmas associated with the use of other actors such as humanitarian agencies and military forces in the provision of health care. Finally, similar tensions were evident in the four areas of the international political economy of health explored in chapter 7. In all four cases I identified not only a tension between individual needs and the state's perceptions of which needs should be prioritized, but also the important role that external actors such as pharmaceutical companies, donor states and philanthropic foundations play in setting priorities.

In the end, it is clear that health and international relations are interdependent for at least three reasons. First, an individual's health is increasingly dependent on decisions made by a variety of actors operating at a global level. Social, economic and political decisions made at the global level – whether patent regulations under TRIPS, donors' acquiescence to their funds being used for abortion procedures, or the scope of humanitarian access – impact on the individual. The state remains the only filter between the global level and the individual level that is capable of cushioning blows and exploiting opportunities, but it too is capable of causing as much harm as good. Clearly, effective and wealthy states are better able to protect their populations from global forces than less wealthy states, but those forces still impact on both albeit to varying degrees.

Second, analysing the global politics of health gives us a better understanding of the underlying dynamics of global politics itself. Understanding *why* health has received little attention in terms of 'high politics' (Fidler and Gostin 2008), and the impact of the logic of high politics on health, allows us to better understand why certain interests take precedence over others at the global level. Price (2008: 20) argues that what is important to understand about IR is not always the material interests (maximizing wealth and military power) but the 'norms and identities that give those interests value and meaning'. In studying the global politics of health we are able to ascertain what political decisions that concern health are taken for granted, and why some experiences, conditions and expectations are given precedence over others.

Third, we still do not fully understand the relationship between politics and health. Much more work is needed to understand how relationships between the growing number of political actors affect health outcomes and to identify the areas of health that should be considered as causal or intervening factors in relations within states, between states and between states and non-state actors. We have only just started to appreciate how these issues – commonly thought to be firmly in the realm of low politics – impact on the world's economy and its politics, and to acknowledge how global politics shapes the health of billions.

NOTES

Introduction

1 As opposed to 'low politics' – which are matters not immediately associated with the survival of the state, e.g. social and cultural relativist positions.

2 Preventable in this use means *primary prevention* as understood in the discipline of epidemiology (science of disease prevention). Primary prevention involves action that can be taken to prevent the development of a disease in a person who is well and does not (yet) have the disease in question; it can involve immunization, access to nutritional food, clean water and shelter, to quit smoking or access to prophylactic devices in the prevention of sexually transmitted diseases (STDs). Essentially, the figure quoted represents the number of children dying – who need not – based on existing biological, clinical and epidemiological data (Gordis 2004: 6).

3 For the rest of the book I will use the terms 'developing' and 'developed'. My use of these terms is informed by the sources that I have accessed, and by the definition provided by the United Nations (UN) Statistics Division. The UN Statistics Division notes that '[T]here is no established convention for the designation of "developed" and "developing" countries or areas in the United Nations system.' However, the Division designates Africa, Americas (excluding North America), countries emerging from the former Yugoslavia, Caribbean, Central and South America, Asia excluding Japan, and Oceania excluding Australia and New Zealand, as 'developing regions', while North America, Europe, Japan, Australia and New Zealand are categorized as 'developed regions'. Traditionally, Eastern Europe, Russia and former USSR territories are not placed in the developing or developed category (UN Statistics Division 2008).

4 Following the rather strange convention of the discipline I use the capitalized 'International Relations' or 'IR' to refer to the academic discipline and the

lower case 'international relations' to refer to actual relations between states.

5   An exception to this is the recent study by Andrew Price-Smith (2009) *Contagion and Chaos: Disease, Ecology, and National Security in the Era of Globalization*, ch. 7 (Cambridge, Mass: MIT Press).

Chapter 1

1   I borrow these terms from Fidler (2005).
2   To use the terms that define a securitizing discourse by Buzan et al. (1998b).
3   Ken Booth (2007: 326) talks about this problem with those seeking the normative goal of human security. When seeking to promote humanity to key international structures, the argument is often lost the moment it needs to be pointed out *why* humanity should be valued in the same way as other 'traditional' security concerns. The original message is lost at this moment because the referent still remains 'traditional' security concerns.

Chapter 2

1   I acknowledge that there are other international organizations such as UNICEF, UNFPA, UNDP and UNAIDS (see chapter 3) that play important roles in 'global health governance'. WHO was selected because its sole mandate is public health and medicine. Likewise, the World Bank was selected because it is the sole international organization that has contributed the most money to health care programmes.
2   For the purposes of this chapter, and in the remainder of the book, I define donor states as those that donate aid at a higher level than that which they receive; and aid-recipient states as those states that receive a higher proportion of aid than what they may (and most do not) donate themselves.
3   The PASB was originally called the International Sanitary Bureau; the name changed to the PASB in 1924.
4   The Essential Medicines List was, perhaps, third to the Alma Ata Declaration and WHO's first foray into international law through the International Code on Breast Milk Substitutes, the most exciting development of the 1970s for WHO (Taylor 1992). The Essential Medicines List, through statistics and research, compiles the names of drugs (and their pharmaceutical developers) that are essential for treating preventable illnesses. If a drug is on this list, it is not meant to be priced above an affordability threshold. See chapter 7 for further discussion of the List.
5   The states that make up G8 are the United States, United Kingdom, Germany, France, Japan, Italy, Russia and Canada.
6   CEA measure the outcome of an approach in terms of 'natural units' – e.g. number of HIV infections averted or malarial infections prevented. A 'good buy' is one that is cost effective and addresses a large burden of disease (Kumaranayake and Walker 2002: 145), according to the 1993 WDR.

7   Though the specific targets in the eight MDGs were developed from the United
    Nations Millennium Declaration and agreed to by Member States at the Fifty-
    Fifth Assembly of the UNGA (Resolution 55.2). Under the heading 'develop-
    ment and poverty eradication', the Declaration included specific health targets
    that were then adopted into Goals 4, 5 and 6 (UNGA 2000; UN 2007).
8   The WHO regional offices responsible for Africa and South East Asia, in which
    the majority of the world's poor live, account for the largest share of the global
    burden of disease, make up 37% of the world's population, but only spend 2%
    of global resources on health. If we exclude Australia, Japan, New Zealand
    and Republic of Korea from the WHO Western Pacific regional office, it still
    accounts for 24% of the world's population that bears 18% of the global burden
    of disease, and yet accounts for only 2% of the world's health resources (WHO
    2007a: 19). The Region of the Americas and the European Region, excluding
    the OECD countries, represents 12% of the world's population, 11% of the
    global burden of disease and spends less than 5% of global health resources
    (WHO 2007a: 19).

Chapter 3

1   A longer history of the health as a right existed in the delivery of social welfare,
    which emerged in Europe in the nineteenth century (Burnham 2005: 122–125).
    During the Enlightenment period there were particular efforts to provide health
    care for the poor. The social welfare movement was based on the presumption
    that health was a positive tenet for human progress (Risse 1992: 173–178,
    194–195).
2   UNAIDS involves the contributive work of UNHCR, UNICEF, UNDP, WFP,
    UNFPA, UNODC, ILO, UNESCO, WHO and the World Bank.
3   The danger of adolescent girls giving birth is that they are at a higher risk of
    malnutrition, which causes complications during pregnancy, or have a pelvis
    that is not yet mature enough to carry a child – creating a high risk of obstetric
    fistula.
4   It should be noted that the female genital mutilation debate also reflects similar
    arguments. According to Audrey Macklin, the 'question that occupies most
    Western academics when they address female genital mutilation (FGM) is
    whether the nation or international community should tolerate the practice. Yet
    the salient issue for most human rights activitists working from within the
    communities where FGM has been prevalent is not whether, but how, to eradi-
    cate the practice' (Macklin 2006: 207). See also Doyal 1995: 87–92, 200–201;
    Abusharaf 2006: 1–26; Ali 2007: 119–128; Booth 2007: 112–113.
5   One important example of this disagreement is the Mexico City Policy, or
    'Global Gag Rule', which the US Bush Administration used to limit USAID
    funding from NGOs that engaged in abortion-related activities, irrespective
    of whether abortion was legal in the country where the NGO was working
    (BBC 2003). Here, we saw the denial of a reproductive health service and the
    right to self-determination. However, the new Obama Administration issued a

Presidential Executive Order that rescinded the Global Gag Rule on 23 January 2009.

Chapter 4

1 Howard Adelman argues that the total was 1.6 million and that the numbers cannot really be known as many did not report to the UNHCR or other aid agencies, there was spontaneous repatriation, and estimates of deaths from cholera may also affect the total figure (Adelman 2003: 98–99).

2 Fiona Terry further discusses the dilemmas that arise in refusing to acknowledge the genuine fear of even these individuals (2002: 173). To demonstrate this, she refers to the fact that RPF leader and, eventually, President of Rwanda, Paul Kagame was involved in human rights abuses and mass killings too, though not on the scale of the Hutu militias (Terry 2002: 173–174). However, the 1951 Convention states under Article 1F(c) and Article 9 that those engaged in crimes against humanity and war crimes disqualify themselves from the protection of refugee status, which means that Article 33: *non-refoulment* (right not to be returned to country of origin if fearing persecution) may not apply to these individuals (Goodwin-Gill and McAdam 2007).

3 Though it should be noted that MSF employee Rony Brauman (1998: 181) argues that choice is often 'not between a political position and a neutral position but between two political positions: one active and the other by default'.

4 With the notable exception of Macrae (2001), Terry (2002) and Keen (2008).

5 Refugee camps on the Chad border; IDP camps within Darfur.

6 The expulsion of up to fifteen humanitarian agencies from Darfur province after President Oman Al-Bashir was indicted for war crimes and crimes against humanity by the Chief Prosecutor of the ICC in March 2009 is a recent example of the politicization of aid.

7 However, this is debatable. Terry (2002), Dijkzeul and Lynch (2006a) and Weiss (2007) have discussed the tension between needing to provide care, while at the same time making sure that the level of assistance does not dissuade refugees from returning. While Talley et al. (2001) and Spiegel and Qassim (2003) argue that in the case of health care, among other provisions, its quality can actually decline the longer refugees are forced to remain in protracted refugee situations. Of course, the continued presence of refugees in camps because of the continued 'benefit' in terms of the aid economy could be a contributing factor to their decline as they remain past the time when aid money is no longer arriving.

8 Castelli presents a survey finding from a study conducted at an international airport terminal in Europe, where up to 94.5% of European travellers stated that they were ready to eat at least one dangerous item (2004: 2).

Chapter 5

1 The Sphere Project then had Phase II which involved training from 1998 to 2000 and a Phase III that involved dissemination and implementation of the Sphere guidelines for members of Sphere (2000–2003).

2 I should mention here that Weiss also makes an excellent point about how some humanitarians are increasingly viewing their role as political actors, in addition to their traditional one of humanitarians. He describes it as a division between the 'classicists' who continue to uphold the principles of neutrality, impartiality and consent'; and the 'solidarists' who 'side with selected victims, publicly confront hostile governments, advocate partisan public policies in donor states, attempt to skew the distribution of aid resources, and refuse to respect the sovereignty of states' (Weiss 2007: 144). Solidarists, in contrast to classicists, do not view humanitarianism as a 'pure' or neutral exercise – it should be 'ameliorative and address structural problems that foment humanitarian crises in the first place' (Weiss 2007: 145). While I think Weiss's description deserves empirical investigation, I use Slim's appreciation of humanitarian work because he divides it according to (a) the effects of immediate aid and (b) the long-term consequences of aid – which allows me to explore how humanitarian medical assistance impacts on the continuation of war.

3 It should be noted that in Bosnia many hospitals were the target of attacks and the need to treat war injuries (which rose from 22% to 78% between April and November 1992) resulted in almost no preventive health activities being carried out (Toole 1999: 18).

Chapter 6

1 I would like to thank an anonymous reviewer for this point.

2 I would like to thank Christian Enemark for his help on this point.

3 Preventable in this use means *primary prevention* as understood in the discipline of epidemiology (science of disease prevention). Primary prevention involves action that can be taken to prevent the development of a disease in a person who is well and does not (yet) have the disease in question (Gordis 2004: 6).

4 Paul Farmer (1999) has argued that it is important to note that in the developing world many of the REIDs have not 're-emerged' at all – they were always present. But the term 're-emergence' is about their reappearance in the developed world, thus indicating who the real security 'referent' object is.

5 It should be noted that infectious diseases can be divided into two categories – bacterial infections and viral infections. Bacterial infections, such as TB and malaria, can be treated with antibiotics to stem the infection; however, the increase of drug-resistant microbes has led to complications in this area. Viral infections, e.g. AIDS, cannot be treated with antibiotics (Shnayerson and Plotkin 2002).

6   However, McInnes and Lee note that this increased interest has 'not supplanted more traditional concerns' (2006: 7).
7   Ships were classified as 'infected', 'suspected' or 'clean'. Quarantine for passengers on cholera- or plague-infected ships was five days (down from ten) and 'deratization' refers to rat eradication measures on ships (Goodman 1971: 70).
8   The revised IHR classify three types of diseases warranting national surveillance and notification to WHO. The first was defined above in the main text. The second type is a case of disease considered unusual or unexpected with a serious public health impact: smallpox, poliomyelitis, human influenza caused by new subtype, severe acute respiratory syndrome (SARS). The third are the following diseases that have demonstrated the ability to cause serious public health impact and spread rapidly internationally: cholera, pneumonic plague, yellow fever, viral haemorrahagic fevers (Ebola, Lassa, Marburg), West Nile fever, other disease of 'special national or regional concern', e.g. dengue fever, Rift Valley fever and meningococcal disease (WHA 2005: 45).

Chapter 7

1   For a discussion on the evolution of the CEA concept see Lee and Goodman; Kumaranayake and Walker; and McPake, all in Lee et al. (2002).
2   DALYs calculate time lost through premature death and time lived with disability – one DALY can be 'thought of as one lost year of "healthy" life and the measured disease burden is the gap between a population's health status and that of a normative reference population' (Beaglehole and Bonita 2004: 35). A QALY calculation assumes that an additional year of life has the same value 'regardless of the age of the person who receives it, assuming that the different life years are of comparable quality' (Brock 2004: 207).
3   I would like to note that Louisiana Lush presents this argument – however, she also notes that 'powerful corporations are heard more loudly than those of the poor' (2004: 17); and that governments and aid agencies have a responsibility to assist developing states in upscaling their health services.
4   This was further aggravated when the anthrax scares in the US after the 9/11 attack led to the US and Canadian governments pressuring the pharmaceutical company Bayer to provide ciprofloxacin at a substantially reduced cost or face a compulsory licence – civil society organizations questioned why this sense of public emergency did not also exist for HIV sufferers in need of antiretroviral drugs (Loff and Heywood 2002: 627).
5   Brazil and Thailand have both experienced heavy pressure from the US and pharmaceutical company lobbyists not to go into generic drug production. For Brazil's experience see Cohen and Lybecker (2005) and Flanagan and Whiteman (2007); for Thailand's experience see Wilson et al. (1999) and Head (2007).
6   The definition of 'concept of equity' is based on the WHO argument for differential pricing (WHO-WTO 2002; Leach et al. 2005: 156). Differential

pricing means that a company would price its product according to purchasing power. An alternative, perhaps even more effective (considering pharmaceutical companies' resistance to differential pricing), pricing mechanism has been suggested by Pogge (2005); also see Selgelid and Sepers (2006).

7   Remember, the US holds 60% of the pharmaceutical industry, the remainder is in Western Europe and Japan (von Braun and Pugatch 2005); these countries encountered similar problems to the US in attracting human volunteers (Shah 2006: 7, 149).

8   The participant has 'nothing to lose' according to the researcher's evaluation of a patient's participation (Annas 1999b: 321).

REFERENCES

Abusharaf, Rogaia Mustafa (2006) 'Introduction: The Custom in Question', in Abusharaf, Rogaia Mustafa (ed.) *Female Circumcision: Multicultural Perspectives*, Philadelphia: University of Pennsylvania Press.

Adelman, Howard (2003) 'The Use and Abuse of Refugees in Zaire', in Stedman, Stephen John and Fred Tanner (eds.) *Refugee Manipulation: War, Politics and the Abuse of Human Suffering*, Washington: Brookings Institution Press.

Agier, Michel and Francoise Bouchet-Saulnier (2004) 'Humanitarian Spaces: Spaces of Exception', in Weissman, Fabrice (ed.) *In the Shadow of 'Just Wars': Violence, Politics and Humanitarian Action*, London: Hurst & Company, Médecins Sans Frontières.

Aginam, Obijiofor (2004) 'Between Isolationism and Mutual Vulnerability: A South–North Perspective on Global Governance of Epidemics in an Age of Globalization', *Temple Law Review*, 77, 297–312.

Aginam, Obijiofor (2005a) *Global Health Governance*, Toronto: University of Toronto Press.

Aginam, Obijiofor (2005b) 'Globalization of Infectious Diseases, International Law and the World Health Organization: Opportunities for Synergy in Global Governance of Epidemics', *New England Journal of International and Comparative Law*, 11(1), 59–74.

Ahoua, L., A. Tamrat, F. Duroch, R.F. Grais and V. Brown (2006) 'High mortality in an internally displaced population in Ituri, Democratic Republic of Congo, 2005: Results of a rapid assessment under difficult conditions', *Global Public Health*, 1(3), 195–204.

Ali, Ayaan Hirsi (2007) *The Caged Virgin*, London: Pocket Books.

Allan, Richard (2003) 'Medicine for Refugees', *Lancet*, Extreme Medicine, 362, 34–35.

Allen, Arthur (2007) *Vaccine: The Controversial Story of Medicine's Greatest Lifesaver*, New York: W.W. Norton & Company.

Allotey, Pascale and Anthony Zwi (2007) 'Population Movements', in Kawachi, Ichiro and Sarah Wamala (eds.) *Globalization and Health*, Oxford: Oxford University Press.

Anderson, Mary B. (1998) 'You Save My Life Today, But for What Tomorrow?' in Jonathan Moore (ed.) *Hard Choices: Moral Dilemmas in Humanitarian Intervention*, Lanham, MD: Rowman & Littlefield Publishers.

Anderson, Tatum (2008a) 'Battles won against Malaria', *Guardian Weekly*, 3 January.

Anderson, Tatum (2008b) 'Life-saver comes at a price', *Guardian Weekly*, 12 September.

Angell, Marcia (1997) 'The Ethics of Clinical Research in the Third World', *New England Journal of Medicine*, 337(12), 847–849.

Angell, Marcia (2004) *The Truth about the Drug Companies: How They Deceive Us and What to Do About It*, New York: Random House.

Annas, George J. (1999a) 'The Impact of Health Policies on Human Rights: AIDS and TB Control', in Mann, Jonathan M., Sofia Gruskin, Michael A. Grodin and George J. Annas (eds.) *Health and Human Rights: A Reader*, New York: Routledge.

Annas, George J. (1999b) 'Questing for Grails: Duplicity, Betrayal, and Self-Deception in Postmodern Medical Research', in Mann, Jonathan M., Sofia Gruskin, Michael A. Grodin and George J. Annas (eds.) *Health and Human Rights: A Reader*, New York: Routledge.

Annas, George J. and Michael A. Grodin (1999) 'Human Rights and Maternal–Fetal HIV Transmission Prevention Trials in Africa', in Mann, Jonathan M., Sofia Gruskin, Michael A. Grodin and George J. Annas (eds.) *Health and Human Rights: A Reader*, New York: Routledge.

Anon. (2004a) 'An Interview with Lee Jong-Wook', *Harvard International Review*, 26(2), 78–81.

Anon. (2004b) 'Public-Health Preparedness Requires More Than Surveillance', *Lancet*, 364, 1639–1640.

Arcel, Libby T. (1998) 'Sexual Torture of Women as a Weapon of War: The Case of Bosnia–Herzegovina', in Arcel, Libby T. (ed.) *War, Violence, Trauma, and the Coping Process*, Copenhagen: International Rehabilitation Council for Torture Victims.

Arunanondchai, Jutamas and Carsten Fink (2007) 'Trade in Health Services in the ASEAN Region', *Health Promotion International*, 21(1), 59–66.

Asal, Victor, Mitchell Brown and Renee Gibson Figueroa (2008) 'Structure, Empowerment and the Liberalization of Cross-National Abortion Rights', *Politics and Gender*, 4(2), 265–284.

Ashford, Mary-Wynne (2008) 'The Impact of War on Women', in Levy, Barry S. and Victor W. Sidel (eds.) *War and Public Health*, 2nd edn, New York: Oxford University Press.

Attaran, Amir and Lee Gillespie-White (2001) 'Do Patents for Anti-retroviral Drugs Constrain Access to HIV/AIDS Treatment in Africa', *Journal of the American Medical Association*, 286(15), 1886–1892.

Attaran, Amir and Brigitte Granville (2004) 'Who Needs To Do What?' in Attaran, Amir and Brigitte Granville (eds.) *Delivering Essential Medicines*, London: Royal Institute of International Affairs.

Axworthy, Lloyd (2001) 'Human Security and Global Governance: Putting People First', *Global Governance*, 7(1), 19–23.

Aylward, R. Bruce, Arnab Acharya, Sarah England, Mary Agocs and Jennifer Linkins (2003) 'Polio Eradication', in Smith, Richard D., Robert Beaglehole, David Woodward and Nick Drager (eds.) *Global Public Goods for Health: Health Economic and Public Health Perspective*, Oxford: Oxford University Press.

Banatvala, Nicholas and Anthony B. Zwi (2000) 'Public Health and Humanitarian Interventions: Developing the Evidence Base', *British Medical Journal*, 321, 101–105.

Banerji, Debabar (2002) 'Report of the WHO Commission on Macroeconomics and Health: A Critique', *International Journal of Health Services*, 32(4), 733–754.

Barnett, Michael and Jack Snyder (2008) 'The Grand Strategies of Humanitarianism', in Barnett, Michael and Thomas G. Weiss (eds.) *Humanitarianism in Question: Politics, Power and Ethics*, Ithaca: Cornell University Press.

Barnett, Michael and Thomas G. Weiss (2008) 'Humanitarianism: A Brief History of the Present', in Barnett, Michael and Thomas G. Weiss (eds.) *Humanitarianism in Question: Politics, Power and Ethics*, Ithaca: Cornell University Press.

Barnett, Tony (2006) 'A Long-Wave Event. HIV/AIDS, Politics, Governance and "Security": Sundering the Intergenerational Bond?' *International Affairs*, 82(2), 297–313.

Barry, Christian and Kate Raworth (2002) 'Access to Medicines and the Rhetoric of Responsibility', *Ethics and International Affairs*, 16(2), 57–70.

Beaglehole, Robert (2005) 'Viewpoints: Global Partnerships for Health', *European Journal of Public Health*, 15(2), 113.

Beaglehole, Robert and Ruth Bonita (2004) *Public Health at the Crossroads: Achievements and Prospects*, Cambridge: Cambridge University Press.

Beiser, Morton (2005) 'The Health of Immigrants and Refugees in Canada', *Canadian Journal of Public Health*, 96(2), 30–44.

Bellamy, Alex J. (2006) *Just Wars: From Cicero to Iraq*, Cambridge: Polity Press.

Benatar, Solmon R. (2003) 'Improving Global Health: The Need to Think "Outside the Box"!', *Monash Bioethics Review*, 22(2), 69–72.

Billson, Janet Mancini (2006) 'The Complexities of Defining Female Well-Being', in Billson, Janet Mancini and Carolyn Fluehr-Lobban (eds.) *Female Well-Being: Toward a Global Theory of Social Change*, London: Zed Books.

Bingham, Nick and Steve Hinchliffe (2008) 'Mapping the Multiplicities of Biosecurity', in Lakoff, Andrew and Stephen J. Collier (eds.) *Biosecurity Interventions: Global Health and Security in Question*, New York: Columbia University Press.

Birn, Anne-Emanuelle (2005) 'Gates's Grandest Challenge: Transcending Technology as Public Health Ideology', *Lancet*, 366, 514–519.

Blouin, Chantal (2007) 'Can the World Trade Organization Help Achieve the Health Millenium Development Goals?' in Cooper, Andrew F., John J. Kirton and Ted Schrecker (eds.) *Governing Global Health: Challenge, Response, Innovation*, Aldershot: Ashgate.

Bonita, Ruth, Alec Irwin and Robert Beaglehole (2007) 'Promoting Public Health in the Twenty-First Century: The Role of the World Health Organization', in Kawachi, Ichiro and Sarah Wamala (eds.) *Globalization and Health*, Oxford: Oxford University Press.

Boone, Catherine and Jake Batnoll (2007) 'Politics and AIDS in Africa: Research Agendas in Political Science and International Relations', in Ostergard, Robert L. Jr. (ed.) *HIV/AIDS and the Threat to National and International Security*, Basingstoke: Palgrave Macmillan.

Booth, Ken (1996) '75 Years on: Rewriting the Subject's Past – Reinventing its Future', in Smith, Steve, Ken Booth and Marysia Zalewski (eds.) *International Theory: Positivism and Beyond*, Cambridge: Cambridge University Press.

Booth, Ken (2005) 'Beyond Critical Security Studies', in Booth, K. (ed.), *Critical Security Studies and World Politics*, Boulder: Lynne Rienner.

Booth, Ken (2007) *Theory of World Security*, Cambridge: Cambridge University Press.

Bower, Jennifer and Peter Chalk (2003) *The Global Threat of New and Reemerging Infectious Disease: Reconciling US National Security and Public Health Policy*, Arlington: RAND Science and Technology.

Brauman, Rony (1998), 'Refugee Camps, Population Transfers, and NGOs', in Jonathan Moore (ed.) *Hard Choices: Moral Dilemmas in Humanitarian Intervention*, Lanham, MD: Rowman & Littlefield Publishers.

Breman, Anna and Carolyn Shelton (2007) 'Structural Adjustment Programs and Health', in Kawachi, Ichiro and Sarah Wamala (eds.) *Globalization and Health*, Oxford: Oxford University Press.

Bristol, Nellie (2006) 'Military Incursions into Aid Work Anger Humanitarian Groups', *Lancet*, 384, 384–386.

BBC (2003) 'US abortion rule "hits Africa women"', 26 September 2003. http:www.newsvote.bbc.co.uk/mpapps/pagetools/print/news.bbc.co.uk/2/hi/africa/3139120.

BBC (2008) 'French aid worker killed in Chad', 1 May 2008. http://news.bbc.co.uk/2/hi/africa/7378304.stm (accessed 20 June 2008).

Brock, Dan W. (2004) 'Ethical Issues in the Use of Cost Effectiveness Analysis for the Prioritisation of Health Care Resources', in Anand, Sudhir, Fabienne Peter and Amartya Sen (eds.) *Public Health, Ethics and Equity*, New York: Oxford University Press.

Brody, Baruch A. (2002) 'Philosophical Reflections on Clinical Trials in Developing Countries' in Rhodes, Rosamond, Margaret P. Battin and Anita Silvers (eds.) *Medicine and Social Justice: Essays on the Distribution of Health Care*, New York: Oxford University Press.

Brown, Hannah (2007) 'Worsening Security in Darfur Could Reverse Health Gains', *Lancet*, 369, 630–632.

Brown, Theodore M., Marcos Cueto and Elizabeth Fee (2006) 'The World Health Organization and the Transition from International to Global Public Health', *American Journal of Public Health*, 96(1), 62–72.

Brundtland, Gro Harlem (2003) 'Global Health and International Security', *Global Governance*, 9, 417–423.

Buchanan, Allen and Matthew Decamp (2006) 'Responsibility for Global Health', *Theoretical Medicine and Bioethics*, 27, 95–114.

Buckup, Sebastian (2008) 'Global Public–Private Partnerships Against Neglected Diseases: Building Governance Structures for Effective Outcomes', *Health Economics, Policy and Law*, 3(1), 31–50.

Bull, Hedley (1977) *The Anarchical Society: A Study of Order in World Politics*, London: Macmillan.

Burci, Gian Luca (2007) 'Health and Infectious Disease', in Weiss, Thomas G. and Sam Daws (eds.) *The Oxford Handbook on the United Nations*, Oxford: Oxford University Press.

Burnett, Angela and Michael Peel (2001) 'Asylum Seekers and Refugees in Britain: Health Needs of Asylum Seekers and Refugees', *British Medical Journal*, 322, 544–547.

Burnham, John C. (2005) *What is Medical History?* Cambridge: Polity Press.

Burns, William (2006) 'Openness is Key in Fight Against Disease Outbreaks', *Bulletin of the World Health Organization*, 84(10), 769–770.

Buse, Kent and Gill Walt (2000a) 'Global Public–Private Partnerships: part I – a new development in health?', *Bulletin of the World Health Organization*, 78(4), 549–561.

Buse, Kent and Gill Walt (2000b) 'Global Public–Private Partnerships: part II – what are the health issues for global governance?', *Bulletin of the World Health Organization*, 78(5), 699–709.

Buse, Kent and Gill Walt (2002) 'Globalization and Multilateral Public–Private Health Partnerships: Issues for Health Policy', in Lee, Kelley, Kent Buse and Suzanne Fustukian (eds.) *Health Policy in a Globalising World*, Cambridge: Cambridge University Press.

Buse, Kent, Nick Drager, Suzanne Fustukian and Kelley Lee (2002) 'Globalisation and Health Policy: Trends and Opportunities', in Lee, Kelley, Kent Buse and Suzanne Fustukian (eds.) *Health Policy in a Globalising World*, Cambridge: Cambridge University Press.

Buse, Kent, Adriane Martin-Hilber, Ninuk Widyantoro and Sarah J Hawkes (2006) 'Management of the Politics of Evidence-Based Sexual and Reproductive Health Policy', *Lancet*, 368, 2101–2103.

Buzan, Barry, David Held and Anthony McGrew (1998a) 'Realism versus Cosmopolitanism', *Review of International Studies*, 24, 387–398.

Buzan, Barry, Ole Weaver and Jaap de Wilde (1998b) *Security: A New Framework for Analysis*, Boulder: Lynne Rienner.

Cahill, Kevin M. (ed.) (1999) *A Framework for Survival: Health, Human Rights and Humanitarian Assistance in Conflicts and Disasters*, 2nd edn, London: Routledge.

Calain, Philippe (2007) 'Exploring the International Arena of Global Health Surveillance', *Health Policy and Planning*, 22(1), 2–12.

Carballo, Manuel (2001) 'Emerging Health Challenges in the Context of Migration', in van Krieken, Peter J. (ed.) *Health, Migration and Return: A Handbook for a Multidisciplinary Approach*, The Hague: T.M.C. Asser Press.

Carballo, Manuel, Jose Julio Divino and Damir Zeric (1998) 'Migration and Health in the European Union', *Tropical Medicine and International Health*, 3(12), 936–944.

Carlin, John (2008) 'War Against Malaria' *Guardian Weekly*, 29 February, 27 29.

Carpenter, Mick (2000) 'Health for Some: Global Health and Social Development since Alma Ata', *Community Development Journal*, 35(4), 336–351.

Carvalho, Simon and Mark Zacher (2001) 'The International Health Regulations in Historical Perspective', in Price-Smith, Andrew T. (ed.) *Plagues and Politics: Infectious Disease and International Policy*, Basingstoke: Palgrave Macmillan.

Cash, Richard A. and Vasant Narasimhan (2000) 'Impediments to Global Surveillance of Infectious Diseases: Consequences of Open Reporting in a Global Economy', *Bulletin of the World Health Organization*, 78(11), 1358–1367.

Castelli, Francesco (2004) 'Human Mobility and Disease: A Global Challenge', *Journal of Travel Medicine*, 11(1), 1–2.

Caulford, Paul and Yasmin Vali (2006) 'Providing Health Care to Medically Uninsured Immigrants and Refugees', *Canadian Medical Association Journal*, 174(9), 1253–1254.

Cawthorne, Paul, Nathan Ford, Jiraporn Limpananont, Nimit Tienudom and Wirat Purahon (2007) 'WHO Must Defend Patients' Interests, not Industry', *Lancet*, 369, 974–975.

Chalk, Peter (2006) 'Disease and the Complex Processes of Securitization in the Asia-Pacific', in Cabarello-Anthony, Mely and Amitav Acharya (eds.) *Non-Traditional Security in Asia: Dilemmas in Securitization*, Aldershot: Ashgate.

Checkel, Jeffrey T. (1998) 'The Constructivist Turn in International Relations Theory', *World Politics*, 50(2), 324–348.

Chrétien, Jean-Paul, David L. Blazes, Joel C. Gaydos, Sheryl A. Bedno, Rodney L. Coldren, Randall C. Culpepper, et al. (2006) 'Experience of a Global Laboratory Network in Responding to Infectious Disease Epidemics', *Lancet Infectious Diseases*, 6(9), 538–539.

Clapham, Andrew (2006) *Human Rights Obligations of Non-State Actors*, Oxford: Oxford University Press.

Cleland, John, Stan Bernstein, Alex Ezeh, Anibal Faunders, Anna Glasier and Jolene Innis (2006) 'Family Planning: The Unfinished Agenda', *Lancet*, 368, 1810–1827.

Cobey, James C., Annette Flanagin and William H. Foege (1997) 'Effective Humanitarian Aid: Our Only Hope of Intervention in Civil War', in Levy, Barry S. and Victor W. Sidel (eds.) *War and Public Health*, Oxford: Oxford University Press.

Coghlan, Benjamin, Richard J. Brennan, Pascal Ngoy, David Dofara, Brad Otto, Mark Clements and Tony Stewart (2006) 'Mortality in the Democratic Republic of Congo: A Nationwide Survey', *Lancet*, 367, 44–51.

Coghlan, Benjamin, Pascal Ngoy, Flavien Mulumba, Colleen Hardy, Valerie Nkamgang Bemo, Tony Stewart, Jennifer Lewis and Richard Brennan (2008) *Mortality in the Democratic Republic of Congo: An Ongoing Crisis*, New York: International Rescue Committee, Melbourne: Burnett Institute. http://www.theirc.org/resources/2007/2006-7_congomortalitysurvey.pdf (accessed 1 August 2008).

Cohen, Jillian Clare and Kristina M. Lybecker (2005) 'AIDS Policy and Pharmaceutical Patents: Brazil's Strategy to Safeguard Public Health', *World Economy*, 28(2), 211–230.

Cohen, Jillian Clare, Patricia Illingworth and Udo Schuklenk (2006) 'Introduction', in Cohen, Jillian Clare, Patricia Illingworth and Udo Schuklenk (eds.) *The Power of Pills: Social, Ethical and Legal Issues in Drug Development, Marketing, and Pricing*, London: Pluto Press.

Cohen, Roberta (2007) 'Response to Hathaway', *Journal of Refugee Studies*, 20(3), 370–376.

Collier, Stephen J. and Andrew Lakoff (2008) 'The Problem of Security Health', in Lakoff, Andrew and Stephen J. Collier (eds.) *Biosecurity Interventions: Global Health and Security in Question*, New York: Columbia University Press.

Collins, Steve (1993) 'The Need for Adult Therapeutic Care in Emergency Feeding Programs: Lessons From Somalia', *Journal of the American Medical Association*, 270(5), 637–638.

Commission on Social Determinants of Health (CSDH) (2008) *Closing the Gap in a Generation: Health Equity through Action on the Social Determinants of Health: Final Report of the Commission on Social Determinants of Health*, Geneva: WHO.

Commonwealth of Australia (2006a) *Being Prepared for an Influenza Pandemic*, Department of Industry, Tourism and Resources. http://www.industry.gov.au/pandemicbusinesscontinuity/ (accessed 3 August 2006).

Commonwealth of Australia (2006b) *Exercise Cumpston '06*. Department of Health and Aging. http://www.health.gov.au/internet/wcms/publishing.nsf/Content/ohp-cumpston.htm (accessed 3 August 2006).

Connell, John (ed.) (2008) *The International Migration of Health Workers*, London: Routledge.

Conroy, Anne C., Justin C. Malewezi, Bizwick Mwale and Richard Pendame (2004) 'Responding to Health Crises: The Frustration of a Small African Country', in Amir, Attaran and Brigitte Granville (eds.) *Delivering Essential Medicines*, London: Royal Institute of International Affairs.

Cook, Rebecca J., Bernard M. Dickens and Mahmoud F. Fathalla (2003) *Reproductive Health and Human Rights: Integrating Medicine, Ethics and Law*, Oxford: Clarendon Press.

Cookson, Susan, Ronald Waldman, Brian Gushulak, Douglas MacPherson, Frederick Burkle, Chirstophe Paquet, Erich Kliewer and Patricia Walker (1998)

'Immigrant and Refugee Health', *Emerging Infectious Diseases*, 4(3), 427–428.

Cooper, Andrew F., John J. Kirton and Ted Schrecker (2007) 'Toward Innovation in Global Health Governance', in Cooper, Andrew F., John J. Kirton and Ted Schrecker (eds.) *Governing Global Health: Challenge, Response, Innovation*, Aldershot: Ashgate.

Cornia, Giovanni Andrea (2001) 'Globalization and Health: Results and Options', *Bulletin of the World Health Organization*, 79(9), 834–841.

Cottingham, Jane and Cynthia Myntti (2003) 'Reproductive Health: Conceptual Mapping and Evidence' in Sen, Gita, Asha George and Piroska Ostlin (eds.) *Engendering International Health*, Cambridge, MA: MIT Press.

Crisp, Jeff (2007) 'Humanitarian Action and Coordination', in Weiss, Thomas G. and Sam Daws (eds.) *The Oxford Handbook on the United Nations*, Oxford: Oxford University Press.

Crooks, Glenna M. (2005) 'The Rights of Patients to Participate in Clinical Research', in Santoro, Michael A. and Thomas M. Gorrie (eds.) *Ethics and the Pharmaceutical Industry*, New York: Cambridge University Press.

Cullet, Philippe (2003) 'Patents and Medicines: The Relationship between TRIPS and the Human Right to Health', *International Affairs*, 79(1), 139–160.

Culyer, Anthony J. and Adam Wagstaff (1993) 'Equity and Equality in Health Care', *Journal of Health Economics*, 12(4), 431–457.

Curci, Gionathan and Massimo Vittori (2004) 'Improving Access to Life-Saving Patented Drugs', *Journal of World Intellectual Property*, 7(5), 739–760.

David, Marcella (2001) 'Rubber Helmets: The Certain Pitfalls of Marshalling Security Council Resources to Combat AIDS in Africa', *Human Rights Quarterly*, 23(3), 560–582.

Davidson, Natasha, S. Skull, G. Chaney, A. Frydenberg, D. Isaacs, P. Kelly, B. Lampropoulos, S. Raman, D. Silcove, J. Buttery, M. Smith, Z. Steel and D. Burgner (2004) 'Comprehensive Health Assessment for Newly Arrived Refugee Children in Australia', *Journal of Paediatrics and Child's Health*, 40(9–10), 565–568.

Davies, Sara E. (2008) 'Securitizing Infectious Disease', *International Affairs*, 84(2), 295–313.

De Cock, Kevin M and Anne M Johnson (1998) 'From Exceptionalism to Normalisation: A Reappraisal of Attitudes and Practice around HIV Testing', *British Medical Journal*, 316, 290–293.

de Waal, Alex (1989) *Famine that Kills: Darfur, Sudan, 1984–1985*, Oxford: Clarendon Press.

de Waal, Alex (1997) *Famine Crimes: Politics and the Disaster Relief Industry in Africa*, London: International African Institute and James Currey.

de Waal, Alex (2006) *AIDS and Power: Why There is No Political Crisis – Yet*, London: Zed Books, International African Institute and Royal African Society.

de Waal, Alex (2007) 'Darfur and the Failure of the Responsibility to Protect', *International Affairs*, 83(6), 1039–1054.

de Zulueta, Paquita (2001) 'Randomized Placebo-Controlled Trials and HIV-Infected Pregnant Women in Developing Countries: Ethical Imperialism or Unethical Exploitation', *Bioethics*, 15(4), 289–311.

Deely, Sean (2005) 'War, Health and Recovery', in Barakat, Sutlan (ed.) *After the Conflict: Reconstruction and Development in the Aftermath of War*, London: I.B. Tauris.

Deshpande, Prabhakar (2005) 'Earn Big Bucks via Health Tourism', *Knight Ridder Tribune Business News*, 27 May.

Diallo, Khassoum (2004) 'Data on the Migration of Health-Care Workers: Sources, Uses, and Challenges', *Bulletin of the World Health Organization*, 82(8), 601–607.

Diamond, Jared (2005) *Guns, Germs and Steel: A Short History of Everybody for the Last 13,000 Years*, London: Vintage.

Dickersin, Kay and Drummond Rennie (2003) 'Registering Clinical Trials', *Journal of the American Medical Association*, 290(4), 516–523.

Dietrich, John W. (2007) 'The Politics of PEPFAR: The President's Emergency Plan for AIDS Relief', *Ethics and International Affairs*, 21(3), 277–291.

Dijkzeul, Dennis and Caroline A. Lynch (2006a) 'NGO Management and Health Care Financing Approaches in the Eastern Democratic Republic of the Congo', *Global Public Health*, 1(2), 157–172.

Dijkzeul, Dennis and Caroline Lynch (2006b) *Supporting Local Health Care in a Chronic Crisis: Management and Financing Approaches in the Eastern Democratic Republic of the Congo*, Washington DC: National Academies Press.

Djeddah, Carol (1995) 'Refugee Families', *World Health*, 48(6), 10–11.

Djeddah, Carol (1996) 'Children and Armed Conflict', *World Health*, 49(6), 12–14.

Djolov, George G. (2004) 'Market Power and the Pharmaceutical Industry in South Africa', *Institute of Economic Affairs*, June, 47–51.

Donnelly, Jack (2003) *Universal Human Rights in Theory and Practice*, 2nd edn, Ithaca: Cornell University Press.

Dorrington, Rob, Leigh Johnson, Debbie Bradshaw and Timothy-John Daniel (2006) *The Demographic Impact of HIV/AIDS in South Africa: National and Provincial Indicators for 2006*, Cape Town: Centre for Actuarial Research, South African Medical Research Council and Actuarial Society of South Africa. http://www.commerce.uct.ac.za/Research_Units/CARE/RESEARCH/ReportsWorkingPapers.asp (accessed 1 July 2008).

Doyal, Lesley (1995) *What Makes Women Sick: Gender and the Political Economy of Health*, Basingstoke: Macmillan Press.

Doyal, Lesley (2005) 'Understanding Gender, Health and Globalization: Opportunities and Challenges', in Kickbusch, Illona, Kari A. Harwig and Justin M. List (eds.) *Globalization, Women and Health in the 21st Century*, New York: Palgrave Macmillan.

Duffield, Mark (2001) *Global Governance and the New Wars: The Merging of Development and Security*, London: Zed Books.

Dupont, Alan (2001) *HIV/AIDS: A Major International Issue*, Asia Pacific Ministerial Meeting 9–10 October 2001, Australian Government Overseas Aid Program. http://www.ausaid.gov.au/publications/pdf/security.pdf (accessed 16 February 2006).

Dyer, Nicole (2002) 'Disease Stalks Afghan Refugees', *Science World*, 58(5), 4–5.

Economist (1998) 'Repositioning the WHO', *The Economist*, 347(8067), 79–81.

Economist (2006) 'Leaders: Less Mary Poppins; Global health', *The Economist*, 381(8503), 14.

Economist (2007) 'WHO's counting? AIDS', *The Economist*, 385(8556), 82.

Economist (2008) 'The side-effects of doing good', *The Economist*, 386(8568), 74.

Elbe, Stefan (2006) 'Should HIV/AIDS Be Securitized? The Ethical Dilemmas of Linking HIV/AIDS and Security', *International Studies Quarterly*, 50(1), 119–144.

Enemark, Christian (2006) 'Pandemic Pending', *Australian Journal of International Affairs*, 60(1), 43–49.

Enemark, Christian (2007) *Disease and Security: Natural Plagues and Biological Weapons in East Asia*, London: Routledge.

FAO, OIE, WHO, UNSIC, UNICEF and The World Bank (2008) *Contributing to One World, One Health: A Strategic Framework for Reducing Risks of Infectious Diseases at the Animal-Human-Ecosystems Interface*, 14 October. Presented at the International Ministerial Conference on Avian and Pandemic Influenza, Sharm el-Sheikh, Egypt, 25–26 October 2008.

Farley, John (2004) *To Cast Out Disease: A History of the International Health Division of the Rockefeller Foundation (1913–1951)*, Oxford: Oxford University Press.

Farmer, Paul (1999) *Infections and Inequality: The Modern Plagues*, Berkeley: University of California Press.

Farmer, Paul (2005) *Pathologies of Power: Health, Human Rights and the New War on the Poor*, Berkeley: University of California Press.

Fassil, Yohannes (2000) 'Looking After the Health of Refugees', *British Medical Journal*, 321, 59.

Fathalla, Mahmoud F., Steven W. Sinding, Allan Rosenfield and Mohammed M.F. Fathalla (2006) 'Sexual and Reproductive Health for All: A Call for Action', *Lancet*, 368, 2095–2100.

Fearnley, Lyle (2008) 'Redesigning Syndromic Surveillance for Biosecurity', in Lakoff, Andrew and Stephen J. Collier (eds.) *Biosecurity Interventions: Global Health and Security in Question*, New York: Columbia University Press.

Feldbaum, Harley and Kelley Lee (2004) 'Public Health and Security', in Ingram, Alan (ed.) *Health, Foreign Policy and Security: Towards a Conceptual Framework for Research and Policy*, London: Nuffield Trust, UK Global Health Programme.

Ferrinho, Paulo, Maria Carolina Omar, Maria de Jesus Fernandes, Pierre Blaise, Ana Margarida Bugalho and Wim Van Lerberghe (2004) 'Pilfering for Survival:

How Health Workers Use Access to Drugs as a Coping Strategy', *Human Resources for Health*, 2(1), 4–10.

Fidler, David P. (1999) *International Law and Infectious Diseases*, Oxford: Clarendon Press.

Fidler, David P. (2003a) 'Antimicrobial Resistance: A Challenge for Global Health Governance', in Lee, Kelley (ed.) *Health Impacts of Globalization: Towards Global Governance*, Basingstoke: Palgrave Macmillan.

Fidler, David P. (2003b) 'Emerging Trends in International Law Concerning Global Infectious Disease Control', *Emerging Infectious Diseases*, 9(3), 285–290.

Fidler, David P. (2003c) 'SARS: Political Pathology of the First Post-Westphalian Pathogen', *Journal of Law, Medicine and Ethics*, 31(4), 485–505.

Fidler, David. P. (2004a) 'Germs, Governance, and Global Public Health in the Wake of SARS', *Journal of Clinical Investigation*, 113(6), 799–804.

Fidler, David P. (2004b) 'Constitutional Outlines of Public Health's "New World Order" ', *Temple Law Review*, 77(2), 247–290.

Fidler, David P. (2004c) *SARS, Governance and the Globalization of Disease*, Basingstoke: Palgrave Macmillan.

Fidler, David P. (2005) 'From International Sanitary Conventions to Global Health Security: The New International Health Regulations', *Chinese Journal of International Law*, 4(2), 325–392.

Fidler, David P. (2007a) 'Architecture amidst Anarchy: Global Health's Quest for Governance', *Global Health Governance*, 1(1), 1–17.

Fidler, David P. (2007b) 'A Pathology of Public Health Securitism: Approaching Pandemics as Security Threats' in Cooper, Andrew F., John J. Kriten and Ted Schecher (ed.), *Covering Global Health: Challenge, Response, Innovation*, Aldershot: Ashgate.

Fidler, David P. (2009) 'Vital Signs: Health and Foreign Policy', *World Today*, February, 27–29.

Fidler, David P. and Lawrence O. Gostin (2008) *Biosecurity in the Global Age: Biological Weapons, Public Health and the Rule of Law*, Stanford: Stanford University Press.

Fidler, David P., David L. Heymann, Stephen M. Ostroff and Terry P. O'Brien (1997) 'Emerging and Reemerging Infectious Diseases: Challenges for International, National, and State Law', *International Lawyer*, 31(3), 773–799.

Fidler, David P., Tony D. Perez and Martin S. Cetron (2003) 'International Considerations', in Goodman, Richard A., Mark A. Rothstein, Richard E. Hoffman, Wilfredo Lopez and Gene W. Matthews (eds.) *Law in Public Health Practice*, Oxford: Oxford University Press.

Finnemore, Martha and Kathryn Sikkink (2001) 'Taking Stock: The Constructivist Research Program in International Relations and Comparative Politics', *Annual Review of Political Science*, 4, 391–416.

Fisher, Jill A. (2006) 'Co-ordinating "Ethical" Clinical Trials: The Role of Research Coordinators in the Contract Research Industry', *Sociology of Health and Illness*, 28(6), 678–694.

Flanagan, William and Gail Whiteman (2007) '"AIDS is Not a Business": A Study in Global Corporate Responsibility – Security Access to Low-Cost HIV Medications', *Journal of Business Ethics*, 73, 65–75.

Fleck, Fiona (2003) 'World Trade Organization Finally Agrees Cheap Drugs Deal', *British Medical Journal*, 327, 517.

Foege, William H. (2006) 'Blurring the Lines: Public and Private Partnerships Addressing Global Health', in Santoro, Michael A. and Thomas M. Gorrie (eds.) *Ethics and the Pharmaceutical Industry*, New York: Cambridge University Press.

Ford, Nathan (2004) 'Patents, Access to Medicines and the Role of Non Governmental Organizations', *Journal of Generic Medicines*, 1(2), 137–145.

Forman, Lisa (2007) 'Trade Rules, Intellectual Property, and the Right to Health', *Ethics and International Affairs*, 21(3), 337–357.

Forsythe, David P. (2005) *The Humanitarians: The International Committee of the Red Cross*, Cambridge: Cambridge University Press.

Freedman, Lynn P. (1999a) 'Censorship and Manipulation of Family Planning Information: An Issue of Human Rights and Women's Health', in Mann, Jonathan M., Sofia Gruskin, Michael A. Grodin and George J. Annas (eds.) *Health and Human Rights: A Reader*, New York: Routledge.

Freedman, Lynn P. (1999b) 'Reflections on Emerging Frameworks of Health and Human Rights', in Mann, Jonathan M., Sofia Gruskin, Michael A. Grodin and George J. Annas (eds.) *Health and Human Rights: A Reader*, New York: Routledge.

Freeman, Robert A. (2006) 'Industry Perspectives on Equity, Access, and Corporate Social Responsibility: A View from the Inside', in Cohen, Jillian Clare, Patricia Illingworth and Udo Schuklenk (eds.) *The Power of Pills: Social, Ethical and Legal Issues in Drug Development, Marketing, and Pricing*, London: Pluto Press.

Frenk, Julio, Octavio Gomez-Dantes, Orvill Adams and Emmanuela E. Gakidou (2001) 'The Globalisation of Health Care', in McKee, Martin, Paul Garner and Robin Stott (eds.), *International Co-operation in Health*, Oxford: Oxford University Press.

Friedman, Matthew J., Peter G. Warfe and Gladys K. Mwiti (2003) 'UN Peacekeepers and Civilian Field Personnel', in Green, Bonnie L., Matthew J. Friedman, Joop T.V.M. de Jong, Susan D. Solomon, Terence M. Keane, John A. Fairbank, et al. (eds.) *Trauma Interventions in War and Peace: Prevention, Practice, and Policy*, New York: Kluwer Academic.

Garfield, Richard M. and Alfred I. Neugut (1997) 'The Human Consequences of War', in Levy, Barry S. and Victor W. Sidel (eds.) *War and Public Health*, New York: Oxford University Press.

Garrett, Laurie (1996) 'The Return of Infectious Disease', *Foreign Affairs*, 75(1), 66–79.

Garrett, Laurie (2001) *Betrayal of Trust: The Collapse of Global Public Health*, Oxford: Oxford University Press.

Garrett, Laurie (2007) 'The Challenge of Global Health', *Foreign Affairs*, 86(1), 14–38.

George, Alexander L. and Andrew Bennett (2005) *Case Studies and Theory Development in the Social Sciences*, Cambridge, MA: MIT Press.

George, Rose (2008) 'Send in the Latrines', *New York Times*, 19 May. http://www.nytimes.com/2008/05/19/opinion/19george.html.

Germov, John (1999) 'Imagining Health Problems as Social Issues', in Germov, John (ed.) *Second Opinion: An Introduction to Health Sociology*, 2nd edn., Melbourne: Oxford University Press.

Ghobarah, Hazem Adam, Paul Huth and Bruce Russett (2004) 'Comparative Public Health: The Political Economy of Human Misery and Well-Being', *International Studies Quarterly*, 48(1), 73–94.

Gillies, Rowan, Tido von Schoen-Angerer and Ellen 't Hoen (2006) 'Historic opportunity for WHO to re-assert leadership', *Lancet*, 368, 1405–1406.

Glasier, Anna and A. Metin Gulmezoglu (2006) 'Putting Sexual and Reproductive Health on the Agenda', *Lancet*, 368, 1550–1551.

Glasier, Anna, A. Metin Gulmezoglu, George P. Schmid, Claudia Garcia Moreno and Paul F.A. Van Look (2006) 'Sexual and Reproductive Health: A Matter of Life and Death', *Lancet*, 368, 1595–1607.

Godlee, Fiona (1994) 'The World Health Organisation: WHO in crisis', *British Medical Journal*, 309, 1424–1428.

Goodman, Neville M. (1971) *International Health Organizations and Their Work*, 2nd edn, Edinburgh: Churchill Livingston.

Goodwin-Gill, Guy S. and Jane McAdam (2007) *The Refugee in International Law*, 3rd edn, Oxford: Oxford University Press.

Gordis, Leon (2004) *Epidemiology*, 3rd edn, Philadelphia: Elsevier Saunders.

Gostin, Lawrence. O. (2004) 'Pandemic Influenza: Public Health Preparedness for the Next Global Health Emergency', *Journal of Law, Medicine and Ethics*, 32(4), 565–573.

Gostin, Lawrence O. (2008) 'Why Rich Countries Should Care About the World's Least Healthy People', *Journal of the American Medical Association*, 298(1), 89–92.

Gostin, Lawrence O. and Zita Lazzarini (1997) *Human Rights and Public Health in the AIDS Pandemic*, New York: Oxford University Press.

Gostin, Lawrence and Jonathan Mann (1999) 'Toward the Development of a Human Rights Impact Assessment for the Formulation and Evaluation of Public Health Policies', in Mann, Jonathan M., Sofia Gruskin, Michael A. Grodin and George J. Annas (eds.) *Health and Human Rights: A Reader*, New York: Routledge.

Gould, Robert and Nancy D. Connell (1997) 'The Public Health Effects of Biological Weapons', in Levy, Barry S. and Victor W. Sidel (eds.) *War and Public Health*, New York: Oxford University Press.

Grant, James P. (1997) 'Children, Wars, and the Responsibility of the International Community', in Levy, Barry S. and Victor W. Sidel (eds.) *War and Public Health*, New York: Oxford University Press.

Grein, Thomas W., Kande-Bure O. Kamara, Guénaël Rodier, Aileen J. Plant, Patrick Bovier, Michael J. Ryan, Takaaki Ohyama and David L. Heymann

(2000) 'Rumors of Disease in the Global Village: Outbreak Verification', *Emerging Infectious Diseases*, 6(2), 97–102.

Gross, Michael L. (2006) *Bioethics and Armed Conflict: Moral Dilemmas of Medicine and War*, Cambridge, Mass: MIT Press.

Gruskin, Sophia (2004) 'Is There a Government in the Cockpit: A Passenger's Perspective or Global Public Health: The Role of Human Rights', *Temple Law Review*, 77(2), 313–334.

Gruskin, Sophia and Daniel Tarantola (2005) 'Health and Human Rights', in Gruskin, Sophia, Michael A. Grodin, George J. Annas and Stephen P. Marks (eds.) *Perspective on Health and Human Rights*, New York: Routledge.

Gruskin, Sophia, Michael A. Grodin, George J. Annas and Stephen P. Marks (2005) 'The Links Between Health and Human Rights', in Gruskin, Sophia, Michael A. Grodin, George J. Annas and Stephen P. Marks (eds.) *Perspective on Health and Human Rights*, New York: Routledge.

Gruskin, Sofia, Edward J Mills and Daniel Tarantola (2007) 'History, Principles, and practice of health and human rights', *The Lancet* 370, 4 August, 449–55.

Gumbo, Perege (2009) 'Africa-IMF Summit Wants Bailout Strategy for Africa', *IPP Media*, 12 March. http://www.ippmedia.com/ipp/guardian/2009/03/12/133223.html (accessed 13 March 2009).

Gushulak, Brian (2001) 'Health Determinants in Migrants: The Impact of Population Mobility on Health', in van Krieken, Peter J. (ed.) *Health, Migration and Return: A Handbook for a Multidisciplinary Approach*, The Hague: T.M.C. Asser Press.

Gustafson, Per, Victor F. Gomes, Cesaltina S. Vieira, Henrik Jensen, Remonie Seng, Renee Norberg, Badara Samb, Anders Naucler and Peter Aaby (2001) 'Tuberculosis Mortality During a Civil War in Guinea-Bissau', *Journal of the American Medical Association*, 286(5), 599–603.

Gwatkin, Davidson R. (1997) 'Global Burden of Disease', *Lancet*, 350, 141.

Haines, Andy, Richard Horton and Zulfiqar Bhutta (2007) 'Primary Health Care Comes of Age. Looking Forward to the 30th anniversary of Alma-Ata: call for papers', *Lancet*, 370, 911–913.

Halliday, Fred (1996) 'The Future of International Relations: Fears and Hopes', in Smith, Steve, Ken Booth and Marysia Zalewski (eds.) *International Theory: Positivism and Beyond*, Cambridge: Cambridge University Press.

Harrell-Bond, Barbara E. (1986) *Imposing Aid: Emergency Assistance to Refugees*, Oxford: Oxford University Press.

Harris, Paul G. and Patricia Siplon (2001) 'International Obligation and Human Health: Evolving Policy Responses to HIV/AIDS', *Ethics and International Affairs*, 15(2), 29–52.

Harrison, M. (2004) *Disease and the Modern World: 1500 to the Present Day*, Cambridge: Polity Press.

Hartcher, Peter and John Garnaut (2006) 'Bird Flu Threatens Misery for Millions', *Sydney Morning Herald*, 16 February. http://www.smh.com.au/news/national/bird-flu-threatens-misery-for-millions/2006/02 (accessed 16 February 2006).

Harvey, Ken (2004) 'Patents, Pills and Politics: The Australia–United States Free Trade Agreement and the Pharmaceutical Benefits Scheme', *Australian Health Review*, 28(2), 218–227.

Hathaway, James (2005) *The Rights of Refugees Under International Law*, Cambridge: Cambridge University Press.

Head, Jonathan (2007) 'Thailand Takes on Drugs Giants', BBC, 26 April. http://newsvote.bbc.co.uk/mpapps/pagetools/print/news.bbc.co.uk/2/hi/asia-pacific/65 (accessed 27 April 2007).

Heaton, Annie (2004) 'Joint Public–Private Initiatives and Developing-Country Health Systems', in Amir, Attaran and Brigitte Granville (eds.) *Delivering Essential Medicines*, London: Royal Institute of International Affairs.

Hestermeyer, Holger P. (2007) 'Canadian-made Drugs for Rwanda: The First Application of the WTO Waiver on Patents and Medicines', *ASIL Insight International Economic Law Edition*, 11, 28. http://www.asil.org/insights/2007/12/insights071210.html (accessed 27 February 2008).

Heymann, David L. (1996) 'Controlling Epidemic Diseases', *World Health*, 6, 9–10.

Heymann, David L. (2002) 'The Microbial Threat in Fragile Times: Balancing Known and Unknown Risks', *Bulletin of the World Health Organization*, 82(3), 179.

Heymann, David L. (2003) 'Evolving Infectious Disease Threats to National and Global Security' in Chen, Lincoln, Jennifer Leaning and Vasant Narasimhan (eds.) *Global Health Challenges for Human Security*, Cambridge, Mass.: Global Equity Initiative, Asia Center and Harvard University. Distributed by Harvard University Press.

Heymann, David L. (2005) 'Dealing with Global Infectious Disease Emergencies', in Gunn, S.W.A., P.B. Mansourian, A.M. Davies, A.Piel and B. McA. Sayers (eds.) *Understanding the Global Dimensions of Health*, New York: Springer, International Association for Humanitarian Medicine Brock Chisholm.

Heymann, David L. and Guenael Rodier (2004) 'Global Surveillance, National Surveillance, and SARS', *Emerging Infectious Diseases*, 10(2), 173.

Higer, Amy J. (1999) 'International Women's Activism and the 1994 Cairo Population Conference', in Meyer, Mary K. And Elisabeth Prugl (eds.) *Gender Politics in Global Governance*, Lanham, MD: Rowman & Littlefield Publishers.

High Level Panel on Threats, Challenges and Change (2004) *A More Secure World: Our Shared Responsibility*, New York: United Nations.

Hill, Kenneth, Kevin Thomas, Carla AbouZahr, Neff Walker, Lale Say, Mie Inoue, Emi Suzuki (2007) 'Estimates of Maternal Mortality Worldwide Between 1990 and 2005: An Assessment of Available Data', *Lancet*, 370, 1311–1319.

Holdstock, Douglas (2001) 'Morbidity and Mortality Among Soldiers and Civilians', in Taipale, Ilkka, P. Helena Makela, Kati Juva, Vappu Taipale, Sergei Kolesnikov, Raj Mutalik and Michael Christ (eds.) *War or Health? A Reader*, London: Zed Books.

Holmes, Alison and James H. Maguire (2000) 'Diseases of Immigrants', in Strickland, G. Thomas (ed.) *Hunter's Tropical Medicine and Emerging Infectious Diseases*, 8th edn, Philadelphia: W.B. Saunders Company.

Horton, Richard (2003) *Health Wars: On the Global Front Lines of Modern Medicines*, New York: New York Review Books.

Horton, Richard (2006) 'A Prescription for AIDS 2006–10', *Lancet*, 368, 716–718.

Howson, Christopher, Harvey Fineberg and Barry Bloom (1998) 'The Pursuit of Global Health: The Relevance of Engagement for Developed Countries' *Lancet*, 351, 586–590.

Hunt, Paul (2003) 'Neglected Diseases, Social Justice and Human Rights: Some Preliminary Observations', *Health and Human Rights Working Paper Series No 4*, Geneva: World Health Organization. http://www.who.int/hhr/working_paper4_neglected%20diseases.pdf (accessed 1 July 2008).

Hunt, Paul (2007) 'Right to the Highest Attainable Standard of Health', *Lancet*, 370, 369–371.

Hyatt, Raymond R. (2007) 'Military Spending: Global Health Threat or Global Public Good?' in Kawachi, Ichiro and Sarah Wamala (eds.) *Globalization and Health*, Oxford: Oxford University Press.

Hyndman, Jennifer (2000) *Managing Displacement: Refugees and the Politics of Humanitarianism*, Minneapolis: University of Minnesota Press.

Institute of Medicine (1992) *Emerging Infections: Microbial Threats to Health in the United States*, Washington: National Academies Press.

International Conference on Population and Development (ICPD) (1994) Programme of Action of the International Conference on Population and Development, United Nations Population Fund. http://www.unfpa.org/icpd/icpd-programme.cfm (accessed 1 July 2008).

International Rescue Committee (IRC) (2006) 'Distributions of Foreign Aid $US Per Capita', *The Congo Crisis at a Glance: The Forgotten Emergency*. http://www.theirc.org/resources/DRC-Slide2-Distributions-Fo.jpg (accessed 16 January 2008).

Iqbal, Zaryab (2006) 'Health and Human Security: The Public Health Impact of Violent Conflict', *International Studies Quarterly*, 50, 631–649.

Jackson, Suzanne E., Fran Perkins, Erika Khandor, Lauren Cordwell, Stephen Hamann and Supakorn Buasai (2007) 'Integrated Health Promotion Strategies: A Contribution to Tackling Current and Future Health Challenges', *Health Promotion International*, 21(1), 75–83.

Jones, Seth G., Lee H. Hilborne, C. Ross Anthony, Lois M. Davis, Federico Girosi, Cheryl Benard, Rachel M. Swanger, Anita Datar Garten and Anga Timilsina (2006) *Securing Health: Lessons from Nation-Building Missions*, Arlington: RAND Corporation.

Kaldor, Mary (2006) *New and Old Wars: Organized Violence in a Global Era*, 2nd edn, Cambridge: Polity Press.

Kallings, Lars O. (2008) 'The First Postmodern Pandemic: 25 years of HIV/AIDS', *Journal of International Medicine*, 263(3), 218–243.

Kaufmann, Judith (2006) 'Intellectual Property Rights and the Pharmaceutical Industry', in Kaufmann, Judith (ed.) *Focus on Intellectual Property Rights*, Washington: US Department of State, Bureau of International Information Programs.

Keen, David (2008) *Complex Emergencies*, Cambridge: Polity Press.

Kelle, Alexander (2007) 'Securitization of International Public Health: Implications for Global Health Governance and the Biological Weapons Prohibition Regime', *Global Governance*, 13, 217–235.

Kelly, Lisa M. and Rebecca J. Cook (2007) 'Book Review: Learning to Dance: Advancing women's reproductive health and well being from the perspectives of public health and human rights', *Global Public Health*, 2(1), 99–102.

Kickbusch, Ilona (2003) 'Global Health Governance: Some Theoretical Considerations on the New Political Space', in Lee, Kelley (ed.) *Health Impacts of Globalization: Towards Global Governance*, Basingstoke: Palgrave Macmillan.

Kickbusch, Ilona (2004) 'The Leavell Lecture – The end of public health as we know it: constructing global public health in the 21st century', *Promotion and Education*, 11(4), 206–213.

Kickbusch, Ilona (2007) 'Responding to the Health Society', *Health Promotion International*, 22(2), 89–91.

Kim, Jim Yong, Aaron Shakow, Arachu Castro, Chris Vanderwarker and Paul Farmer (2003) 'Tuberculosis Control', in Smith, Richard, Robert Beaglehole, David Woodward and Nick Drager (eds.) *Global Public Goods for Health: Health Economic and Public Health Perspectives*, Oxford: Oxford University Press.

Kimball, Ann Marie (2006) *Risky Trade: Infectious Disease in the Era of Global Trade*, Aldershot: Ashgate.

Kindhauser, Mary Kay (ed.) (2003) *Communicable Diseases 2002: Global Defence Against the Infectious Disease Threat*, WHO/CDS/2003.15, Geneva: World Health Organization.

Kirby, Michael (1996) 'Human Rights and the HIV Paradox', *Lancet*, 348, 1217–1218.

Kirton, John J. and Ella Kokotsis (2007) 'Keeping Faith with Africa's Health: Catalysing G8 Compliance', in Cooper, Andrew F., John J. Kirton and Ted Schrecker (eds.) *Governing Global Health: Challenge, Response, Innovation*, Aldershot: Ashgate.

Knudsen, Lara M. (2006) *Reproductive Rights in a Global Context: South Africa, Uganda, Peru, Denmark, United States, Vietnam, Jordan*, Nashville: Vanderbilt University Press.

Koivusalo, Meri and Eeva Ollila (1997) *Making a Healthy World: Agencies, Actors and Policies in International Health*, Helsinki: Stakes, London: Zed Books.

Kongolo, Tshimanga (2001) 'Public Interest versus the Pharmaceutical Industry's Monopoly in South Africa', *Journal of World Intellectual Property*, 4(5), 609–627.

Konttinen, Mauno (2001) 'Postwar Health and Health Care in Bosnia and Herzegovina', in Taipale, Ilkka, P. Helena Makela, Kati Juva, Vappu Taipale,

Sergei Kolesnikov, Raj Mutalik and Michael Christ (eds.) *War or Health? A Reader*, London: Zed Books.

Kumaranayake, Lilani (2006) 'Global Governance of International Public Health: The Role of International Regulatory Cooperation', in Roberts, Jennifer A. (ed.) *The Economics of Infectious Disease*, Oxford: Oxford University Press.

Kumaranayake, Lilani and Sally Lake (2002) 'Regulation in the Context of Global Health Markets', in Lee, Kelley, Kent Buse and Suzanne Fustukian (eds.) *Health Policy in a Globalising World*, Cambridge: Cambridge University Press.

Kumaranayake, Lilani and Damian Walker (2002) 'Cost-effectiveness Analysis and Priority-Setting: Global Approach without Local Meaning?' in Lee, Kelley, Kent Buse and Suzanne Fustukian (eds.) *Health Policy in a Globalising World*, Cambridge: Cambridge University Press.

Kuwahara, Steven S. (2007) 'Outsourcing Insights: Understand the Pros and Cons of Outsourcing to Developing Countries', *Biopharm International*, 20(2), 30–32.

Labonte, Ronald (2001) 'Health Promotion in the 21st Century: Celebrating the Ordinary', *Health Promotion Journal of Australia*, 11(2), 104–109.

Labonte, Ronald and Ted Schrecker (2007) 'Foreign Policy Matters: A Normative View of the G8 and Population Health', *Bulletin of the World Health Organization*, 85(3), 185–191.

Lakoff, Andrew (2008) 'From Population to Vital System: National Security and the Changing Object of Public Health' in Lakoff, Andrew and Stephen H Collier (eds.) *Biosecurity Interventions: Global Health and Security in Question*, New York: Columbia University Press.

Lancet (2002) 'Patently robbing the poor to serve the rich', *Lancet*, 360, 885.

Lancet (2006) 'Migration and health: a complex relation', *Lancet*, 368, 1039.

Lancet (2007a) 'Making abortion legal, safe and rare', *The Lancet*, 370, 28 July, 291.

Lancet (2007b) 'Science at WHO and UNICEF: the corrosion of trust', *The Lancet*, 370, 22 September, 1007.

Lavergne, Marc and Fabrice Weissman (2004) 'Sudan: Who Benefits from Humanitarian Aid?' in Weissman, Fabrice (ed.) *In the Shadow of 'Just Wars': Violence, Politics and Humanitarian Action*, London: Hurst & Company, Médecins Sans Frontières.

Leach, Beryl, Joan E. Paluzzi and Paula Munderi (2005) *Prescription for Healthy Development: Increasing Access to Medicines*, London: Earthscan, United Nations Development Programme.

Leaning, Jennifer (1999a) 'Introduction', in Leaning, Jennifer, Susan M. Briggs and Lincoln C. Chen (eds.) *Humanitarian Crises: The Medical and Public Health Response*, Cambridge, Mass: Harvard University Press.

Leaning, Jennifer (1999b) 'Emergency Care', in Leaning, Jennifer, Susan M. Briggs and Lincoln C. Chen (eds.) *Humanitarian Crises: The Medical and Public Health Response*, Cambrdige, Mass: Harvard University Press.

Leaning, Jennifer, Susan M. Briggs and Lincoln C. Chen (eds.) (1999) *Humanitarian Crises: The Medical and Public Health Response*, Cambridge, Mass: Harvard University Press.

Lee, Jong-Wha and Warwick J. McKibbin (2003) 'Globalization and Disease: The Case of SARS', *Working Papers in International Economics No. 5.03*, Sydney: Lowry Institute for International Policy.

Lee, Kelley (2003) *Globalization and Health: An Introduction*, Basingstoke: Palgrave Macmillan.

Lee, Kelley (2009) *The World Health Organization*, Routledge Global Institutions, Oxford: Routledge.

Lee, Kelley and Hilary Goodman (2002) 'Global Policy Networks: The Propagation of Health Care Financing Reform since the 1980s', in Lee, Kelley, Kent Buse and Suzanne Fustukian (eds.) *Health Policy in a Globalising World*, Cambridge: Cambridge University Press.

Lee, Kelley and Richard Dodgson (2003) 'Globalization and Cholera: Implications for Global Governance', in Lee, Kelley (ed.) *Health Impacts of Globalization: Towards Global Governance*, Basingstoke: Palgrave Macmillan.

Lee, Kelley and Colin J. McInnes (2003) 'Health, Foreign Policy and Security: A Discussion Paper', *UK Global Health Programme Working Paper No. 1*, London: Nuffield Trust.

Lee, Kelley and Anthony Zwi (2003) 'A Global Political Economy Approach to AIDS: Ideology, Interests and Implications', in Lee, Kelley (ed.) *Health Impacts of Globalization: Towards Global Governance*, Basingstoke: Palgrave Macmillan.

Lee, Kelley, Kent Buse and Suzanne Fustukian (eds.) (2002) *Health Policy in a Globalising World*, Cambridge: Cambridge University Press.

Levy, Barry S. and Victor W. Sidel (1997) 'Preventing War and Its Health Consequences: Roles of Public Health Professionals', in Levy, Barry S. and Victor W. Sidel (eds.) *War and Public Health*, New York: Oxford University Press.

Lewis, Stephen (2005) *Race Against Time: Searching for Hope in AIDS-Ravaged Africa*, Toronto: House of Anansi Press.

Lieu, Tracy A., Thomas G. McGuire and Alan R. Hinman (2005) 'Overcoming Economic Barriers to the Optimal Use of Vaccines', *Health Affairs*, 24(3), 666–680.

Lippert, Owen (2002) 'A Market Perspective on Recent Developments in the TRIPS and Essential Medicines Debate', in Granville, Brigitte (ed.) *The Economics of Essential Medicines*, London: Royal Institute of International Affairs.

Lischer, Sarah Kenyon (2005) *Dangerous Sanctuaries: Refugee Camps, Civil War, and the Dilemmas of Humanitarian Aid*, Ithaca: Cornell University Press.

Litsios, Socrates (2004) 'Primary Health Care, WHO and the NGO Community', *Development*, 47(2), 57–63.

Loff, Bebe and Mark Heywood (2002) 'Patents on Drugs: Manufacturing Scarcity or Advancing Health?' *Journal of Law, Medicine and Ethics*, 30(4), 621–631.

Low, Nicola, Nathalie Broutet, Yaw Adu-Sarkodie, Pelham Barton, Mazeda Hossain and Sarah Hawkes (2006) 'Global Control of Sexually Transmitted Infections', *Lancet*, 368, 2001–2016.

Lu, Chunling, Catherine M. Michaud, Emmanuela Gakidou, Kashif Khan and Christopher J.L. Murray (2006) 'Effect of the Global Alliance for Vaccines and Immunisation on Diphtheria, Tetanus, and Pertussis Vaccine Coverage: an Independent Assessment', *Lancet*, 368, 1088–1095.

Luna, Florencia (2006) 'Assumptions in the Standard of Care Debate', in Cohen, Jillian Clare, Patricia Illingworth and Udo Schuklenk (eds.) *The Power of Pills: Social, Ethical and Legal Issues in Drug Development, Marketing, and Pricing*, London: Pluto Press.

Lurie, Peter and Sidney M. Wolfe (1997) 'Unethical Trials of Interventions to Reduce Perinatal Transmission of Human Immunodeficiency Virus in Developing Countries', *New England Journal of Medicine*, 337(12), 853–856.

Lush, Louisiana (2002) 'The International Effort for Anti-Retrovirals: Politics or Public Health?' in Granville, Brigitte (ed.) *The Economics of Essential Medicines*, London: Royal Institute of International Affairs, International Economics Programme.

Lush, Louisiana (2004) 'Why Do the Poor Lack Access to Essential Medicines' in Attaran, Amir and Brigitte Granville (eds.) *Delivering Essential Medicines*, London: Royal Institute of International Affairs.

Lush, Louisiana and Oona Campbell (2001) 'International Co-operation for Reproductive Health: Too Much Ideology?' in McKee, Martin, Paul Garner and Robin Stott (eds.) *International Co-operation in Health*, Oxford: Oxford University Press.

MacDonald, Rhona (2007) 'Access to Essential Medicines and the Pendulum of Power', *Lancet*, 369, 983–984.

Mack, Eric (2006) 'The World Health Organization's New International Health Regulations: Incursions on State Sovereignty and Ill-fated Response to Global Health Issues', *Chicago Journal of International Law*, 7(1), 365–377.

Macklin, Audrey (2006) 'The Double-Edged Sword: Using the Criminal Law Against Female Genital Mutilation in Canada', in Abusharaf, Rogaia Mustafa (ed.) *Female Circumcision: Multicultural Perspectives*, Philadelphia: University of Pennsylvania Press.

MacNaughton, Gillian (2004) 'Women's Human Rights Related to Health-Care Services in the Context of HIV/AIDS', *Health and Human Rights Working Paper Series No 5*, Geneva: World Health Organization. http://www.who.int/hhr/information/papers/en/index.html (accessed 1 July 2008).

Macrae, Joanna (2001) *Aiding Recovery? The Crisis of Aid in Chronic Political Emergencies*, London: Zed Books, Overseas Development Institute.

MacReady, Norra (2007) 'Developing Countries Court Medical Tourists', *Lancet*, 369, 1849–1850.

Malaysia Ministry of Health (2007) Malaysia Healthcare. http://www.myhealthcare.gov.my/ (accessed 23 August 2009).

Malkki, Lisa (1995) 'Refugees and Exile: From "Refugee Studies" to the National Order of Things', *Annual Review of Anthropology*, 24, 495–523.

Manciaux, M. and T.M. Fliedner (2005), 'World Health: A Mobilizing Utopia?' in Gunn, S.W.A., P.B. Mansourian, A.M. Davies, A.Piel and B.

McA. Sayers (eds.), *Understanding the Global Dimensions of Health*, New York: Springer, International Association for Humanitarian Medicine Brock Chisholm.

Mann, Jonathan M. (1999) 'Human Rights and AIDS: The Future of a Pandemic', in Mann, Jonathan M., Sofia Gruskin, Michael A. Grodin and George J. Annas (eds.) *Health and Human Rights: A Reader*, New York: Routledge.

Mann, Jonathan M. and Daniel Tarantola (1998) 'Responding to HIV/AIDS: A Historical Perspective, 2', *Health and Human Rights*, 2(4), 5–8.

Mann, Jonathan M., Lawrence Gostin, Sofia Gruskin, Troyen Brennan, Zita Lazzarini and Harvey Fineberg (1999), 'Health and Human Rights', in Mann, Jonathan M., Sofia Gruskin, Michael A. Grodin and George J. Annas (eds.) *Health and Human Rights: A Reader*, New York: Routledge.

McCarthy, Michael (2007) 'The Global Fund: 5 Years On', *Lancet*, 370, 307–308.

McCoy, David, Ravi Narayan, Fran Baum, David Sanders, Hani Serag, Jane Salvage, et al. (2006) 'A New Director-General for WHO – An Opportunity for Bold and Inspirational Leadership', *Lancet*, 368, p.2179–2183.

McGinn, Therese and K. Allen (2006) 'Improving Refugees' Reproductive Health through Literacy in Guinea', *Global Public Health*, 1(3), 229–248.

McGuinness, Margaret E. (2003) 'Legal and Normative Dimensions of the Manipulation of Refugees', in Stedman, Stephen John and Fred Tanner (eds.) *Refugee Manipulation: War, Politics and the Abuse of Human Suffering*, Washington: Brookings Institution Press.

McInnes, Colin J. (2004) 'Health and Foreign Policy', in Ingram, Alan (ed.) *Health, Foreign Policy and Security: Towards a Conceptual Framework for Research and Policy*, London: Nuffield Trust, UK Global Health Programme.

McInnes, Colin J. and Kelley Lee (2006) 'Health, Security and Foreign Policy', *Review of International Studies*, 32(1), 5–23.

McMichael, Anthony J. and R. Beaglehole (2000) 'The Changing Global Context of Public Health', *Lancet*, 356, 495–499.

McMichael, Anthony J. and Colin D. Butler (2007) 'Emerging Health Issues: The Widening Challenge for Population Health Promotion', *Health Promotion International*, 21(1), 15–24.

McNeil, Donald G. (2008) 'Gates Foundation's Influence Criticized', *New York Times*, 16 February. http://www.nytimes.com/2008/02/16/science/16malaria.html (accessed 12 March 2008).

McNeill, William H. (1998) *Plagues and Peoples*, 3rd edn, New York: Anchor Books.

McPake, Barbara (2002) 'The Globalization of Health Sector Reform Policies: Is "Lesson Drawing" Part of the Process?' in Lee, Kelley, Kent Buse and Suzanne Fustukian (eds.) *Health Policy in a Globalising World*, Cambridge: Cambridge University Press.

Médecins Sans Frontières (MSF) (1997) *Refugee Health: An Approach to Emergency Situations*, Oxford: Macmillan.

Melrose, Dianna (1982) *Bitter Pills: Medicines and the Third World Poor*, Oxford, Oxfam.

Menken, Jane and M. Omar Rahman (2006) 'Reproductive Health', in Merson, Michael H., Robert E. Black and Anne J. Mills (eds.) *International Public Health: Diseases, Programs, Systems and Policies*, 2nd edn, Boston: Jones & Bartlett Publishers.

Mi rinnnn, Angela and Malik Peiris (2005) 'International Health Regulations (2005)', *Lancet*, 366, 1249 1261.

Messiant, Christine (2004) 'Angola: Woe to the Vanquished', in Weissman Fabrice (ed.) *In the Shadow of 'Just Wars': Violence, Politics and Humanitarian Action*, London: Hurst & Company, Médecins Sans Frontières.

Mjones, Staffan (2005) 'Refugee Children – A Concern for European Paediatricians', *European Journal of Paediatrics*, 164, 535–538.

Murray, Christopher J.L. (1994) 'Quantifying the Burden of Disease: The Technical Basis for Disability-Adjusted Life Years', *Bulletin of the World Health Organization*, 72, 495–509.

Murray, Christopher J.L., Thomas Laakso, Kenji Shibuya, Kenneth Hill and Alan D. Lopez (2007), 'Can We Achieve Millennium Development Goal 4? New analysis of country trends and forecasts of under-5 mortality to 2015', *Lancet*, 370, 1040–1054.

Murray, Sally B. and Sue A. Skull (2005) 'Hurdles to Health: Immigrant and Refugee Health Care in Australia', *Australian Health Review*, 29(1), 25–29.

Musgrove, Philip (2000) 'A Critical Review of "A Critical Review": The Methodology of the 1993 World Development Report', *Health Policy and Planning*, 15(1), 110–115.

Mytelka, Lynn K. (2006) 'Pathways and Policies to (Bio) Pharmaceutical Innovation Systems in Developing Countries', *Industry and Innovation*, 13(4), 415–435.

Nakaya, Sumie (2004) 'Women and Gender Equality in Peacebuilding: Somalia and Mozambique', in Keating, Tom and W. Andy Knight (eds.) *Building Sustainable Peace*, Alberta: University of Alberta Press and Tokyo: United Nations University Press.

Nambiar, Ravi (2004) 'KPJ Gears Up to Tap Buoyant Health Tourism Market', *Business Times*, New Straits Times Press, 1 September.

Nanda, Priya (2006) 'I Would Pay, if I Could Pay in Maize: Trade Liberalization, User Fees in Health and Women's Health Seeking in Tanzania', in Grown, Caren, Elissa Braunstein and Anju Malhotra (eds.) *Trading Women's Health and Rights?* London: Zed Books.

Nathaniel, Pramodh (2003) 'Limiting the Spread of Communicable Diseases Caused by Human Population Movement', *Journal of Rural and Remote Environmental Health*, 2(1), 23–32.

Navarro, Vicente (1999) 'Health and Equity in the World in the Era of "Globalization"', *International Journal of Health Services*, 29(2), 215–226.

Nettleton, Sarah (2006) *The Sociology of Health and Illness*, 2nd edn., Cambridge: Polity Press.

Ngwena, Charles (2004) 'An Appraisal of Abortion Laws in Southern Africa from a Reproductive Health Rights Perspective', *Journal of Law, Medicine and Ethics*, 32(4), 708–717.

Nogues, Julio J. (1993) 'Social Costs and Benefits of Introducing Patent Protection for Pharmaceutical Drugs in Developing Countries', *Developing Economies*, 31(1), 24–53.

Noji, Eric K. and Brent T. Burkholder (1999) 'Public Health Interventions', in Leaning, Jennifer, Susan M. Briggs and Lincoln C. Chen (eds.) *Humanitarian Crises: The Medical and Public Health Response*, Cambridge, Mass: Harvard University Press.

Nordstrom, Anders (2006) 'What's Next for WHO?' *Lancet*, 368, 177–179.

Nullis-Kapp, Clare (2005) 'Efforts Under Way to Stem "Brain Drain" of Doctors and Nurses', *Bulletin of the World Health Organization*, 83(2), 84–85.

Office of UN Deputy Special Representative of the UN Secretary-General for Sudan, UN Resident and Humanitarian Co-ordinator for Humanitarian Affairs (OCHA) (2007) *Darfur Humanitarian Profile No. 29*, 1 October. http://ochaonline.un.org/sudan/SituationReports/DarfurHumanitarianNeedsProfile/tabid/3368/Default.aspx (accessed 1 July 2008).

Ogata, Sadako and Amartya Sen (2003) *Human Security Now*, Commission on Human Security. http://www.humansecurity-chs.org (accessed 1 July 2008).

Olness, Karen N. (1998) 'Refugee Health', in Loue, Sana (ed.) *Handbook of Immigrant Health*, New York: Plenum Press.

Orbinski, James (2007) 'Global Health, Social Movements, and Governance', in Cooper, Andrew F., John J. Kirton and Ted Schrecker (eds.) *Governing Global Health: Challenge, Response, Innovation*, Aldershot: Ashgate.

Ostergard, Robert L. (2002) 'Politics in the Hot Zone: AIDS and the Threat to Africa's Security', *Third World Quarterly*, 23(2), 333–350.

Palinkas, Lawrence A., Sheila M. Pickwell, Kendra Brandstein, Terry J. Clark, Linda L. Hill, Robert J. Moser and Abdikadir Osman (2003) 'The Journey to Wellness: Stages of Refugee Health Promotion and Disease Prevention', *Journal of Immigrant Health*, 5(1), 19–28.

Palmer, Celia A. and Anthony B. Zwi (1998) 'Women, Health and Humanitarian Aid in Conflict', *Disasters*, 22(3), 236–249.

Pannenborg, Charles O. (1979) *A New International Health Order: An Inquiry into the International Regulations of World Health and Medical Care*, Germantown, MD: Sijthoff & Noordhoff.

Papastergiadis, Nikos (2000) *The Turbulence of Migration: Globalization, Deterritorialization and Hybridity*, Cambridge: Polity Press.

Paris, Roland (2001) 'Human Security: Paradigm Shift or Hot Air?' *International Security*, 26(2), 87–102.

Patel, Preeti and Paolo Tripodi (2007) 'Linking HIV to Peacekeepers', in Ostergard, Robert L. Jr. (ed.) *HIV/AIDS and the Threat to National and International Security*, Basingstoke: Palgrave Macmillan.

People's Health Movement, Medact, Global Equity Gauge Alliance (2005) *Global Health Watch 2005: An Alternative World Health Report*, London: Zed Books, Pretoria: UNISA Press.

Perkins, Anne (2008) 'Time to Review the Millennium Development Goals', *Guardian*, 25 September. http://www.guardian.co.uk/katine/2008/sep/25/aidanddevelopment.news (accessed 1 October 2008).

Perrin, Pierre (1999) 'The Risks of Military Participation', in Leaning, Jennifer, Susan M. Briggs and Lincoln C. Chen (eds.) *Humanitarian Crises: The Medical and Public Health Response, Cambridge, Mass. Harvard University* sity Press.

Peterson, Susan (2006) 'Epidemic Disease and National Security', *Security Studies*, 12(2), 43–81.

Petryna, Adriana (2007) 'Clinical Trials Offshored: On Private Sector Science and Public Health', *BioSocieties*, 2, 21–40.

Petryna, Adriana and Arthur Kleinman (2006) 'The Pharmaceutical Nexus: An Introduction', in Petryna, Adriana, Andrew Lakoff and Arthur Kleinman (eds.) *Global Pharmaceuticals: Ethics, Markets, Practices*, Durham, NC: Duke University Press.

Pirages, Dennis (1997) 'Ecological Theory and International Relations', *International Journal of Global Legal Studies*, 5, 53.

Pogge, Thomas (2002) *World Poverty and Human Rights*, Cambridge: Polity.

Pogge, Thomas (2004) 'Relational Conceptions of Justice: Responsibilities for Health Outcomes', in Anand, Sudhir, Fabienne Peter and Amartya Sen (eds.) *Public Health, Ethics and Equity*, New York: Oxford University Press.

Pogge, Thomas (2005) 'Human Rights and Global Health: A Research Program', *Metaphilosophy*, 36(1/2), 182–209.

Poku, Nana K. (2005) *AIDS in Africa: How the Poor are Dying*, Cambridge: Polity Press.

Poletti, Timothy (2004) 'Cost-Recovery in the Health Sector: An Inappropriate Policy in Complex Emergencies', *Humanitarian Exchange Magazine*, 26, 19–22.

Pollock, Allyson M. and David Price (2003) 'New Deal from the World Trade Organization: May Not Provide Essential Medicines for Poor Countries', *British Medical Journal*, 327, 571–572.

Ponteva, Matti (2001) 'The Impact of Warfare on Medicine', in Taipale, Ilkka, P. Helena Makela, Kati Juva, Vappu Taipale, Sergei Kolesnikov, Raj Mutalik and Michael Christ (eds.) *War or Health? A Reader*, London: Zed Books.

Porter, John, Kelley Lee and Jessica Ogden (2002) 'The Globalization of DOTS: Tuberculosis as a Global Emergency', in Lee, Kelley, Kent Buse and Suzanne Fustukian (eds.) *Health Policy in a Globalising World*, Cambridge: Cambridge University Press.

Potts, Malcolm and Julia Walsh (1999) 'Making Cairo Work', *Lancet*, 353, 315.

Powles, John and Flavio Comim (2003) 'Public Health Infrastructure and Knowledge', in Smith, Richard, Robert Beaglehole, David Woodward and Nick Drager (eds.) *Global Public Goods for Health: Health Economic and Public Health Perspectives*, Oxford: Oxford University Press.

Preker, Alexander S. (2004) 'From Health to Wealth and Back to Health', in Attaran, Amir and Brigitte Granville (eds.) *Delivering Essential Medicines*, London: Royal Institute of International Affairs.

Price, Richard (2008) 'Moral Limit and Possibility in World Politics', in Price, Richard M. (ed.) *Moral Limit and Possibility in World Politics*, Cambridge: Cambridge University Press.

Price-Smith, Andrew T. (2001) 'Introduction', in Price-Smith, Andrew T. (ed.) *Plagues and Politics: Infectious Disease and International Policy*, Basingstoke: Palgrave.

Price-Smith, Andrew T. (2002) *The Health of Nations: Infectious Disease, Environmental Change, and Their Effects on National Security and Development*, Cambridge, Mass.: MIT Press.

Price-Smith, Andrew T. (2009) *Contagion and Chaos: Disease, Ecology, and National Security in the Era of Globalization*, Cambridge, Mass: MIT Press.

R. v Cambridge Health Authority [1995] EWCA Civ 49, 10 March. http://www.bailii.org/ew/cases/EWCA/Civ/1995/49.html (accessed 1 July 2008).

Ramiah, Ilavenil (2006) 'Securitizing the AIDS Issue in Asia', in Caballero-Anthony, Mely and Amitav Acharya (eds.) *Non-Traditional Security in Asia: Dilemmas in Securitization*, Aldershot: Ashgate.

Ranson, M. Kent, Robert Beaglehole, Carlos M. Correa, Zafar Mirza, Kent Buse and Nick Drager (2002) 'The Public Health Implications of Multilateral Trade Agreements', in Lee, Kelley, Kent Buse and Suzanne Fustukian (eds.) *Health Policy in a Globalising World*, Cambridge: Cambridge University Press.

Reed, Shelby D., Robert M. Califf and Kevin A. Schulman (2007) 'Is There a Price to Pay for Short-Term Savings in the Clinical Development of New Pharmaceutical Products?' *Drug Information Journal*, 41(4), 491–499.

Reimann, Kim D. (2006) 'A View from the Top: International Politics, Norms and the Worldwide Growth of NGOs', *International Studies Quarterly*, 50(1), 45–67.

Resnik, David B. (2001) 'Developing Drugs for the Developing World: An Economic, Legal, Moral, and Political Dilemma', *Developing World Bioethics*, 1(1), 11–32.

Reuters AlertNet (2008) 'Darfur Conflict: Peace Elusive as Security Worsens', *Reuters AlertNet*, 15 July. http://www.alertnet.org/db/crisisprofiles/SD_DAR.html (accessed 25 July 2008).

Richards, Tessa (2001) 'New Global Health Fund: Must be Well Managed if it is to Narrow the Gap between Rich and Poor Countries', *British Medical Journal*, 322, 1321–1322.

Richardson, Michael (2006) 'Express Delivery of H5N1 via Migratory Birds', *Australian Journal of International Affairs*, 60(1), 51–58.

Richey, Lisa Ann (2005) 'Uganda: HIV/AIDS and Reproductive Health', in Chavkin, Wendy and Ellen Chesler (eds.) *Where Human Rights Begin: Health, Sexuality and Women in the New Millennium*, New Jersey: Rutgers University Press.

Riddell, Roger C. (2007) *Does Foreign Aid Really Work?* Oxford: Oxford University Press.

Risse, Guenter B. (1992) 'Medicine in the Age of Enlightenment', in Wear, Andrew (ed.) *Medicine in Society: Historical Essays*, Cambridge: Cambridge University Press.

Risse, Thomas, and Kathryn Sikkink (1999) 'The Socialization of International Human Rights Norms into Domestic Practices: Introduction', in Risse, Thomas, Stephen C. Ropp and Kathryn Sikkink (eds.) *The Power of Human Rights: International Norms and Domestic Change*, Cambridge: Cambridge University Press.

Roberts, Jennifer A. (2006) 'Introduction to the Economics of Infectious Disease', in Roberts, Jennifer A. (ed.) *The Economics of Infectious Disease*, Oxford: Oxford University Press.

Roberts, Les and Charles Lubula Muganda (2008) 'War in the Democratic Republic of Congo', in Levy, Barry S. and Victor W. Sidel (eds.) *War and Public Health*, 2nd edn, Oxford: Oxford University Press.

Rodier, Guenael R., Michael J. Ryan and David L. Heymann (2000) 'Global Epidemiology of Infectious Diseases', in Strickland, G. Thomas (ed.) *Hunter's Tropical Medicine and Emerging Infectious Diseases*, 8th edn, Philadelphia: W.B. Saunders Company.

Roth, Cathy (2006) 'Epidemic and Pandemic Alert and Response', *Refugee Survey Quarterly*, 25(4), 10–103.

Ruger, Jennifer P. (2005) 'The Changing Role of the World Bank in Global Health in Historical Perspective', *American Journal of Public Health*, 95(1), 60–70.

Ruger, Jennifer P. (2007) 'Rethinking Equal Access: Agency, Quality and Norms', *Global Public Health*, 2(1), 78–96.

Ruger, Jennifer P. and Derek Yach (2005) 'Global Functions at the World Health Organization', *British Medical Journal*, 330, 1099–1100.

Sachs, Jeffrey D. (2001) *Macroeconomics and Health: Investing in Health for Economic Development*, Report on the Commission on Macroeconomics and Health, Geneva, World Health Organization.

Sachs, Jeffrey D. (2002) 'Investing in Health for Economic Development' in World Health Organization, *Scaling Up Response to Infectious Diseases*, Geneva: World Health Organization.

Sachs, Jeffrey D. and John W. McArthur (2005) 'The Millennium Project: A Plan for Meeting the Millennium Development Goals', *Lancet*, 365, 347–353.

Saker, Lance, Kelley Lee and Barbara Cannito (2007) 'Infectious Disease in the Age of Globalization', in Kawachi, Ichiro and Sarah Wamala (eds.) *Globalization and Health*, Oxford: Oxford University Press.

Salama, Peter, Paul Spiegel and Richard Brennan (2001) 'No Less Vulnerable: The Internally Displaced in Humanitarian Emergencies', *Lancet*, 357, 1430–1431.

Sampath, Padmashree Gehl (2006) 'India's Product Patent Protection Regime: Less or More of "Pills for the Poor"?', *Journal of World Intellectual Property*, 9(6), 694–726.

Sanders, David and Mickey Chopra (2003) 'Globalization and the Challenge of Health for All: A View from Sub-Saharan Africa', in Lee, Kelley (ed.) *Health Impacts of Globalization: Towards Global Governance*, Basingstoke: Palgrave Macmillan.

Santa Barbara, Joanna and Graeme MacQueen (2004) 'Peace Through Health: Key Concepts', *Lancet*, 364, 384–386.

Santoro, Michael A. (2005) 'Charting a Sustainable Path for the Twenty-First Century Pharmaceutical Industry', in Santoro, Michael A. and Thomas M. Gorrie (eds.) *Ethics and the Pharmaceutical Industry*, New York: Cambridge University Press.

Save the Children (2008) *Saving Children's Lives: Why Equity Matters*. http://www.savethechildren.org.uk/en/54_4231.html (accessed 1 July 2008).

Scherer, Frederic M. (2004) 'A Note on Global Welfare in Pharmaceutical Patenting', *World Economy*, 27(7), 1127–1142.

Schrecker, Ted and Ronald Labonte (2007) 'What's Politics Got to Do with It? Health, the G8 and the Global Economy', in Kawachi, Ichiro and Sarah Wamala (eds.) *Globalization and Health*, Oxford: Oxford University Press.

Schrecker, Ted, Ronald Labonte and David Sanders (2007) 'Breaking Faith with Africa: The G8 and Population Health', in Cooper, Andrew F., John J. Kirton and Ted Schrecker (eds.) *Governing Global Health: Challenge, Response, Innovation*, Aldershot: Ashgate.

Schuklenk, Udo (2003) 'Intellectual Property Rights, Compulsory Licensing and the TRIPS Agreement: Some Ethical Issues', *Monash Bioethics Review*, 22(2), 63–68.

Schwartlander, Bernhard, Ian Grubb and Jos Perriens (2006) 'The 10-year Struggle to Provide Antiretroviral Treatment to People with HIV in the Developing World', *Lancet*, 368, 541–546.

Scutchfield, F. Douglas and John M. Last (2003) 'Public Health in North America', in Beaglehole, Robert (ed.) *Global Public Health: A New Era*, Oxford: Oxford University Press.

Seal, Andrew J., Paul I. Creeke, Zahra Mirghani, Fathia Abdalla, Rory P. McBurney, Lisa S. Pratt, Dominique Brookes, Laird J. Ruth and Elodie Marchand (2005) 'Iron and Vitamin A Deficiency in Long-Term African Refugees', *Journal of Nutrition*, 135(4), 808–813.

Sedgh, Gilda, Stanley Henshaw, Susheela Singh, Elisabeth Ahman and Iqbal H Shah (2007) 'Induced Abortion: Estimated Rates and Trends Worldwide', *Lancet*, 370, 1338–1345.

Selgelid, Michael J. and Eline M. Sepers (2006) 'Patents, Profits, and the Price of Pills: Implications for Access and Availability', in Cohen, Jillian Clare, Patricia Illingworth and Udo Schuklenk (eds.) *The Power of Pills: Social, Ethical and*

Legal Issues in Drug Development, Marketing, and Pricing, London: Pluto Press.

Sen, Amartya (2004) 'Why Health Equity?' in Anand, Sudhir, Fabienne Peter and Amartya Sen (eds.) *Public Health, Ethics and Equity*, New York: Oxford University Press.

Sen, Chiranjoy (2005) 'Thai Health Tourism Gives India Headache', *Knight Ridder Tribune Business News*, 27 July.

Senanayake, Pramilla and Susanne Hamm (2004) 'Sexual and Reproductive Health Funding: Donors and Restrictions', *London*, 363, 70

Shadlen, Kenneth (2007) 'The Political Economy of AIDS Treatment: Intellectual Property and the Transformation of Generic Supply', *International Studies Quarterly*, 51(3), 559–581.

Shah, Sonia (2006) *The Body Hunters: Testing New Drugs on the World's Poorest Patients*, New York: New Press.

Shepard, Bonnie (2006) *Running the Obstacle Course to Sexual and Reproductive Health: Lessons from Latin America*, Westport, Connecticut: Praeger.

Shetty, Priya (2007) 'How Important is Neutrality to Humanitarian Aid Agencies?', *Lancet*, 370, 377–378.

Shisana, Olive, Nompumelelo Zungu-Dirwayi and William Shisana (2003) 'AIDS: A Threat to Human Security', in Chen, Lincoln, Jennifer Leaning and Vasant Narasimhan (2003) *Global Health Challenges for Human Security*, Cambridge, Mass.: Global Equity Initiative, Asia Center and Harvard University. Distributed by Harvard University Press.

Shnayerson, Michael and Mark J. Plotkin (2002) *The Killers Within: The Deadly Rise of Drug-Resistant Bacteria*, Boston: Little, Brown & Company.

Siddiqi, Javed (1995) *World Health and World Politics: The World Health Organization and the UN System*, Columbia: University of South Carolina Press.

Sidel, Victor W. (1997) 'The Roles and Ethics of Health Professionals in War', in Levy, Barry S. and Victor W. Sidel (eds.) *War and Public Health*, New York: Oxford University Press.

Sidel, Victor W. and Barry, S. Levy (2001) 'The Health and Social Consequences of Diversion of Economic Resources to War and Preparation for War', in Taipale, Ilkka, P. Helena Makela, Kati Juva, Vappu Taipale, Sergei Kolesnikov, Raj Mutalik and Michael Christ (eds.) *War or Health? A Reader*, London: Zed Books.

Sidel, Victor W. and Barry S. Levy (2003) 'War, Terrorism and Public Health', *Journal of Law, Medicine and Ethics*, 31(4), 516–523.

Siegel, Richard Lewis (1996) 'AIDS and Human Rights', *Human Rights Quarterly*, 18(3), 612–640.

Sikkink, Kathryn (1986) 'Codes of Conduct for Transnational Corporations: The Case of the WHO/UNICEF Code', *International Organization*, 40(4), 815–840.

Simunovic, Vladimir (2007) 'Health Care in Bosnia and Herzegovina Before, During, and After 1992–1995 War: A Personal Testimony', *Conflict and Health*, 1(1), 7–13.

Singer, P. W. (2002) 'AIDS and International Security', *Survival*, 44(1), 145–158.

Singh, Kavita, Unni Karunakara, Gilbert Burnham and Kenneth Hill (2005) 'Forced Migration and Under-Five Mortality: A Comparison of Refugees and Hosts in North-Western Uganda and Southern Sudan', *European Journal of Population*, 21, 247–270.

Slim, Hugo (1997) 'Doing the Right Thing: Relief Agencies, Moral Dilemmas and Moral Responsibility in Political Emergencies and War', *Disasters*, 21(3), 244–257.

Slim, Hugo (2003) 'Why Protect Civilians? Innocence, Immunity and Enmity in War', *International Affairs*, 79(3), 481–501.

Slim, Hugo (2008) *Killing Civilians: Method, Madness, and Morality in War*, New York: Columbia University Press.

Small Arms Survey (2005) *Small Arms Survey 2005: Weapons at War*, New York: Oxford University Press.

Smolinski, Mark S., Margaret A. Hamburg and Joshua Lederberg (2003) (eds.) *Microbial Threats to Health: Emergence, Detection and Response*, Washington: National Academies Press.

Sphere Project (2004) *Sphere Humanitarian Charter and Minimum Standards in Disaster Response*, Sphere Handbook 2004 edition. http://www.sphereproject. org/content/view/146/84/lang,english/ (accessed 2 November 2008).

Spiegel, Paul B. (2004) 'HIV/AIDS Among Conflict-Affected and Displaced Populations: Dispelling Myths and Taking Action', *Disasters*, 28(3), 322–339.

Spiegel, Paul B. and Mohamed Qassim (2003) 'Forgotten Refugees and Other Displaced Populations', *Lancet*, 362, 72–74.

Spiegel, Paul B. and Peter Salama (2000) 'War and Mortality in Kosovo 1998–1999: An Epidemiological Testimony', *Lancet*, 355, 2204–2209.

Spiegel, Paul B., Mani Sheik, Carol Gotway-Crawford and Peter Salama (2002) 'Health Programmes and Policies Associated with Decreased Mortality in Displaced People in Postemergency Phase Camps: A Retrospective Study', *Lancet*, 360, 1927–1934.

Stanwell-Smith, Ros (2003) 'Health of Asylum Seekers and Refugees – The UK's Response', *Health and Hygiene*, 24(3), 4–6.

Starrs, Ann M. (2007) 'Delivering for Women', *Lancet*, 370, 1285–1287.

Stedman, Stephen John and Fred Tanner (2003) 'Refugees as Resources in War', in Stedman, Stephen John and Fred Tanner (eds.) *Refugee Manipulation: War, Politics and the Abuse of Human Suffering*, Washington: Brookings Institution Press.

Stein, Barry N. (1987) 'Economic and Political Considerations Relevant to Refugee Health Care', in Sandler, Richard H. and Thomas C. Jones (eds.) *Medical Care of Refugees*, New York: Oxford University Press.

Stern, Alexandra Minna and Howard Markel (2004) 'International Efforts to Control Infectious Diseases, 1851–Present', *Journal of the American Medical Association*, 292(12), 1474–1479.

Subramanian, Arvind (2004) 'Has the Intellectual Property Pact Opened a Pandora's Box for the Pharmaceuticals Industry?' *Finance and Development*, 41(1), 22–25.

Supari, Siti Fadilah (2008) *It's Time for the World to Change: In the Spirit of Dignity, Equity and Transparency*, Jakarta: PT Sulaksana Watinsa Indonesia.

Talley, Leisel, Paul B. Spiegel and Mona Girgis (2001) 'An Investigation of Increasing Mortality among Congolese Refugees in Lugufu Camp, Tanzania, May–June 1999' *Journal of Refugee Studies*, 14(4), 412–427.

Taylor, Allyn Lise (1992) 'Making the World Health Organization Work: A Legal Framework for Universal Access to the Conditions for Health', *American Journal of Law and Medicine*, 18(4), 301–346.

Taylor, Allyn Lise (1997) 'Controlling the Global Spread of Infectious Diseases: Toward a Reinforced Role for the International Health Regulations', *Houston Law Review*, 33, 1327–1362.

Taylor, Allyn Lise (2002) 'Global Governance, International Health Law and WHO: Looking Towards the Future', *Bulletin of the World Health Organization*, 80(12), 975–980.

Taylor, Allyn Lise (2004) 'Governing the Globalization of Public Health', *Journal of Law, Medicine and Ethics*, 32(3), 500–508.

Taylor, Allyn L., Douglas W. Bettcher and Richard Peck (2003) 'International Law and the International Legislative Process: The WHO Framework Convention on Tobacco Control', in Smith, Richard, Robert Beaglehole, David Woodward and Nick Drager (eds.) *Global Public Goods for Health: Health Economic and Public Health Perspectives*, Oxford: Oxford University Press.

Terry, Fiona (2000) *The Limits and Risks of Regulation Mechanisms for Humanitarian Action*, Humanitarian Exchange No.17, London: Overseas Development Institute.

Terry, Fiona (2002) *Condemned to Repeat? The Paradox of Humanitarian Action*, Ithaca: Cornell University Press.

Terry, Fiona (2004) 'North Korea: Feeding Totalitarianism', in Weissman, Fabrice (ed.) *In the Shadow of 'Just Wars': Violence, Politics and Humanitarian Action*, London: Hurst & Company, Médecins Sans Frontières.

Thakur, Ramesh and Thomas G. Weiss (2009) 'United Nations "policy": an argument with three illustrations', *International Studies Perspectives*, 10(1), 28–35.

Thenabadu, Asoka (2005) 'Spectre of Disease Looms', *Hospital Doctor*, 24 February, 25.

Thomas, Caroline (1989) 'On the Health of International Relations and the International Relations of Health', *Review of International Studies*, 15, 273–280.

Thomas, Caroline (2000) *Global Governance, Development and Human Security*, London: Pluto.

Thomas, Caroline (2003) 'Trade Policy, the Politics of Access to Drugs and Global Governance for Health' in Lee, Kelley (ed.) *Health Impacts of Globalization: Towards Global Governance*, Basingstoke: Palgrave Macmillan.

Thomas, Caroline and Martin Weber (2004) 'The Politics of Global Health Governance: Whatever Happened to "Health for All by the Year 2000"?', *Global Governance*, 10(2), 187–205.

Toebes, Brigit (1999a) *The Right to Health as a Human Right in International Law*, Antwerp: Intersentia-Hart.

Toebes, Brigit (1999b) 'Towards an Improved Understanding of the International Human Right to Health', *Human Rights Quarterly*, 21(3), 661–679.

Tomasevski, Katarina (2005) 'Why a Human Rights Approach to HIV/AIDS Makes All the Difference', *Human Rights and Poverty Reduction Paper*, February, London: Overseas Development Institute. http://www.odi.org.uk/rights/Meeting%20Series/HIVAIDS_HRBA.pdf (accessed 1 July 2008).

Tong, Jacqui (2004) 'Questionable Accountability: MSF and Sphere in 2003', *Disasters*, 28(2), 176–189.

Toole, Michael J. (1999) 'The Role of Rapid Assessment', in Leaning, Jennifer, Susan M. Briggs and Lincoln C. Chen (eds.) *Humanitarian Crises: The Medical and Public Health Response*, Cambridge, Mass: Harvard University Press.

Toole, Michael J. (2000) 'Refugees and Migrants', in Whitman, Jim (ed.) *The Politics of Emerging and Resurgent Infectious Diseases*, Basingstoke: Macmillan Press.

Toole, Michael J. (2003) 'The Health of Refugees: An International Public Health Problem', in Allotey, Pascale (ed.) *The Health of Refugees: Public Health Perspectives from Crisis to Settlement*, Melbourne: Oxford University Press.

Toole, Michael J. (2008) 'Displaced Persons and War', in Levy, Barry S. and Victor W. Sidel (eds.) *War and Public Health*, 2nd edn, New York: Oxford University Press.

Toole, Michael J. and Ronald J. Waldman (1993) 'Refugees and Displaced Persons: War, Hunger, and Public Health', *Journal of the American Medical Association*, 270(5), 600–605.

Toole, Michael J., Ronald J. Waldman and Anthony Zwi (2006) 'Complex Emergencies', in Merson, Michael H., Robert E. Black and Anne J. Mills (eds.) *International Public Health: Diseases, Programs, Systems and Policies*, 2nd edn, Boston: Jones & Bartlett Publishers.

Torres-Cantero, Alberto M., A.G. Miguel, C. Gallardo and S. Ippolito (2007) 'Health Care Provision for Illegal Migrants: May Health Policy Make a Difference?' *European Journal of Public Health*, 17(5), 483–485.

Traub, James (2006) *The Best Intentions: Kofi Annan and the UN in the Era of American Power*, London: Bloomsbury.

Tsafack Temah Chrystelle (2008) 'Gender Discriminations and HIV/AIDS Epidemic in Sub-Saharan Africa', First Prize, *Global Development Network Awards and Medals Competition*, January 2008. http://www.gdnet.org/pdf2/gdn_library/annual_conferences/Ninth_annual_conference/Temah_paper_parallel_session2.4.pdf (accessed 1 July 2008).

Turner, Barry S. (1997) 'Foreword: From Governmentality to Risk, Some Reflections on Foucault's Contribution to Medical Sociology', in Petersen, Alan and Robin Bunton (eds.) *Foucault, Health and Medicine*, London: Routledge.

United Nations (UN) (2007) *The Millennium Development Goals Report 2007*, New York: United Nations.

UNAIDS (2007) *AIDS Epidemic Update: December 2007*, Geneva: UNAIDS and World Health Organization. http://www.unaids.org/en/KnowledgeCentre/HIVData/EpiUpdate/EpiUpdArchive/2007/ (accessed 1 July 2008).

United Nations Children's Emergency Fund (UNICEF) (2008) *The State of the World's Children 2009: Maternal and Newborn Health*, New York: UNICEF, December.

United Nations (UN) Committee on Social, Economic and Cultural Rights (2000) *The Right to the Highest Attainable Standard of Health*, E/C.12/2000/4 (General Comments), 11 August 2000.

United Nations Department of Public Information (2008a) 'Press Conference on Global Campaign for Health Millennium Development Goals', News and Media Division, 25 September. www.un.org/News/briefings/docs//2008/080925_MDG_Health.doc.htm (accessed 26 September 2008).

United Nations Department of Public Information (2008b) 'Secretary-General Calls Record on Maternal Health a Silent Emergency', United Nations Radio, 25 September. www.un.org/apps/news/story.asp?NewsID+28262&Cr=Maternal+Health&Cr1=&Kw1=maternal&Kw2=&Kw3 (accessed 26 September 2008).

United Nations Development Programme (UNDP) (1994) *Human Development Report*, Oxford: Oxford University Press.

UNDP/UNFPA/WHO/World Bank Special Programme of Research, Development and Research Training in Human Reproduction (2004) *Research on Reproductive Health at WHO – Pushing the Frontiers of Knowledge*, Geneva: World Health Organization.

United Nations General Assembly (UNGA) (1948) *Universal Declaration of Human Rights*, New York: United Nations. http://www.un.org/Overview/rights.html (accessed 1 July 2008).

UNGA (1966) *International Covenant on Economic, Social and Cultural Rights*, New York: United Nations. http://www2.ohchr.org/english/law/cescr.html (accessed 1 July 2008).

UNGA (1979) *Convention on the Elimination of All Forms of Discrimination against Women*, Resolution 34/180, 18 December.

UNGA (2000) *United Nations Millennium Declaration*, Resolution 55/2, 18 September.

UNGA (2008) 'Supporting Efforts to End Obstetric Fistula', *Report of the Secretary-General*, Sixty-third session, Item 59 of the provisional agenda, A/63/222, 6 August.

United Nations High Commissioner for Refugees (UNHCR) (2007a) *Convention and Protocol Relating to the Status of Refugees*, Geneva: UNHCR, http://www.unhcr.org/protect/PROTECTION/3b66c2aa10.pdf (accessed 1 July 2008).

UNHCR (2007b) *2006 Global Trends: Refugees, Asylum-seekers, Returnees, Internally Displaced and Stateless Persons*, Division of Operational Services Field Information and Coordination Support Section, Revised July, Geneva: UNHCR.

UNHCR (2008) 'Q&A: Former Health Minister Seeks a Peace Cure for DRC', *UNHCR News Stories*, 25 July. http://www.unhcr.org/news/NEWS/4889d7174. html (accessed 25 July 2008).

United Nations Statistics Division (2008) *Composition of macro geographic (continental) regions, geographic sub-regions, and selected economic and other groupings*, 17 October 2008. http://unstats.un.org/unsd/methods/m49/m49regin. htm#ftnc (accessed 2 March 2009).

USAID (1998) *Reducing the Threat of Infectious Diseases*, Washington: USAID. http://www.usaid.gov/our_work/global_health/id/idstrategy.pdf (accessed 1 July 2008).

United States (US) Department of Defense (DoD) (1998) *Addressing Emerging Infectious-Disease Threats: A Strategic Plan for the Department of Defense*, Washington: DoD Global Emerging Infections Surveillance and Response System.

Usdin, Shereen (2007) *The No-Nonsense Guide to World Health*, Oxford: New Internationalist.

Vande Walle, Gudrun and Paul Ponsaers (2006) 'Formal and Informal Pharmaceutical Economies in Third World Countries: Synergetic, Symbiotic or Parasitical?' *Crime, Law and Social Change*, 45, 361–372.

Vergara, Alfredo E., Joy M. Miller, David R. Martin and Susan T. Cookson (2003) 'A Survey of Refugee Health Assessments in the United States', *Journal of Immigrant Health*, 5(2), 67–73.

von Braun, Johanna and Meir P. Pugatch (2005) 'The Changing Face of the Pharmaceutical Industry and Intellectual Property Rights', *Journal of World Intellectual Property*, 8(5), 599–623.

Waisbord, Silvio (2005) 'Linking Communication for Campaign and Routine Immunization: In Need of a Bifocal View', in Haider, Muhiuddin (ed.) *Global Public Health Communication: Challenges, Perspectives and Strategies*, Boston: Jones & Bartlett Publishers.

Wakabi, Wairagala (2007a) 'Ethnic War Leaves Burundi's Health Sector in Ruins', *Lancet*, 369, 1847–1848.

Wakabi, Wairagala (2007b) 'Health and Humanitarian Situation Worsens in Somalia', *Lancet*, 370, 1201–1202.

Waldman, Ronald J. (2001a) 'Public Health in Times of War and Famine: What Can Be Done? What Should Be Done?' *Journal of the American Medical Association*, 286(5), 588–590.

Waldman, Ronald J. (2001b) 'Prioritising Health Care in Complex Emergencies', *Lancet*, 357, 1427–1429.

Waldman, Ronald J. (2008) 'The Roles of Humanitarian Assistance', in Levy, Barry S. and Victor W. Sidel (eds.) *War and Public Health*, 2nd edn, Oxford: Oxford University Press.

Walker, R.B.J. (1993) *Inside/Outside: International Relations as Political Theory*, Cambridge: Cambridge University Press.

Walker, R.B.J. (1997) 'The Subject of Scrutiny', in Krause, Keith and Michael C. Williams (eds.) *Critical Security Studies: Concepts and Cases*, London: UCL Press.

Walt, Gill and Kent Buse (2006) 'Global Cooperation in International Public Health', in Merson, Michael H., Robert E. Black and Anne J. Mills (eds.) *International Public Health: Diseases, Programs, Systems and Policies*, Boston: Jones & Bartlett Publishers.

Walt, Stephen M. (1991) 'The Renaissance of Security Studies', *International Studies Quarterly*, 35(1), 211–239.

Walt, Kenneth N, (1979) *Theory of International Politics*, London: McGraw-Hill.

Wamala, Sarah, Ichiro Kawachi and Besinati Phiri Mpepo (2007) 'Poverty Reduction Strategy Papers: Bold New Approach to Poverty Eradication or Old Wine in New Bottles?' in Kawachi, Ichiro and Sarah Wamala (eds.) *Globalization and Health*, Oxford: Oxford University Press.

Warkentin, Craig (2002) *Reshaping World Politics: NGOs, the Internet, and Global Civil Society*, Lanham, MD: Rowman & Littlefield Publishers.

Watts, Sheldon (1997) *Epidemics and History: Disease, Power and Imperialism*, New Haven: Yale University Press.

Wechsler, Jill (2006) 'Partnerships Develop New Drugs for Third-World Nations', *Pharmaceutical Technology*, 30(9), 32–42.

Weiss, Thomas G. (2007) *Humanitarian Intervention: Ideas in Action*, Cambridge: Polity Press.

Weiss, Thomas G. and Peter J. Hoffman (2005) 'Making Humanitarianism Work', in Chesterman, Simon, Michael Ignatieff and Ramesh Thakur (eds.) *Making States Work: State Failure and the Crisis of Governance*, Tokyo: United Nations University Press.

Weissman, Fabrice (ed.) (2004) *In the Shadow of 'Just Wars': Violence, Politics and Humanitarian Action*, London: Hurst & Company, in association with Médecins Sans Frontières.

Weston, Elizabeth (1999) 'A Drug by Any Other Name: Brand Power in the Pharmaceutical Industry', *New Doctor*, Spring, 2–11.

White, Hugh (2005) 'More Than a Dose of Flu', *The Age*, 12 September. http://www.theage.com.au/news/hugh-white/more-than-a-dose-of-flu/2005/09/11/112 (accessed 16 February 2006).

Whitman, Jim (2000) 'Political Processes and Infectious Diseases', in Whitman, Jim (ed.) *The Politics of Emerging and Resurgent Infectious Diseases*, Basingstoke: Macmillan Press.

Wight, Colin (2004) 'Theorising the Mechanisms of Conceptual and Semiotic Space', *Philosophy of the Social Sciences*, 34(2), 283–299.

Wilson, David, Paul Cawthorne, Nathan Ford and Saree Aongsonwang (1999) 'Global Trade and Access to Medicines: AIDS Treatments in Thailand', *Lancet*, 354, 1893–1895.

Wipfli, Heather, Douglas W. Bettcher, Chitra Subnramaniam, and Allyn L. Taylor (2001) 'Confronting the Global Tobacco Epidemic: Emerging Mechanisms of Global Governance', in McKee, Martin, Robin Stott and Paul Garner (eds.) *International co-operation in health*, Oxford: Oxford University Press.

Woodruff, Bradley A. (2006) 'Interpreting Mortality Data in Humanitarian Emergencies', *Lancet*, 367, 9–10.

Woodward, David, Nick Drager, Robert Beaglehole and Debra Lipson (2001) 'Globalization and Health: A Framework for Analysis and Action', *Bulletin of the World Health Organization*, 79(9), 875–881.

World Bank (2009) 'Bank Lending, Financial Year "08", Operations. http://www.worldbank.org/wbinfo/lending/lending-home.htm (accessed 15 February 2009).

World Health Assembly (WHA) (2004) *International migration of health personnel: a challenge for health systems in developing countries*, Fifty-Seventh World Health Assembly, WHA Resolution 57.19, 22 May.

WHA (2005) *Revision of the International Health Regulations*, Fifty-Eighth World Health Assembly, A58/4, 16 May.

WHA (2006) *Constitution of the World Health Assembly*, Geneva: World Health Organization.   http://www.who.int/governance/eb/who_constitution_en.pdf (accessed 1 July 2008).

World Health Organization (WHO) (2000a) *A Framework for Global Outbreak Alert and Response*, WHO/CDS/CSR/2000.2, Geneva: WHO Department of Communicable Disease Surveillance and Response.

WHO (2000b) 'Consensus Meeting on Surveillance of Infectious Diseases', Report on a WHO Meeting in Grottaferrata, Italy, 4–7 April, EUR/00/5016367, Copenhagen: WHO Regional Office for Europe, 2000.

WHO (2001) *Macroeconomics and Health: Investing in Health for Economic Development*, Report of the Commission on Macroeconomics and Health, WHO: Geneva. www.cmhealth.org (accessed 3 August 2006).

WHO (2002) *Global Crises – Global Solutions: Managing Public Health Emergencies of International Concern through the revised International Health Regulation*, WHO/CDS/CSR/GAR/2002.4, Geneva: World Health Organisation.

WHO (2005a) *The International Health Regulations (2005)*, Geneva: WHO. http://www.who.int/csr/ihr/current/en (accessed 11 January 2006).

WHO (2005b) 'World Health Assembly Adopts New International Health Regulations: New Rules Govern National and International Response to Disease Outbreaks', 25 May. http://www.who.int/mediacentre/news/releases/2005/pr_wha03/en/print.html (accessed 11 January 2006).

WHO (2006) *Ten things you need to know about pandemic influenza*. http://www.who.int/csr/disease/influenza/pandemic10things/en/index.html (accessed 2 December 2006).

WHO (2007a) *World Health Statistics 2007*, Geneva: World Health Organization.

WHO (2007b) *The World Health Report 2007: A Safer Future: Global Public Health Security in the 21st Century*, Geneva: World Health Organization.

WHO (2007c) *The Global MDR-TB & XDR-TB Response Plan 2007–2008*, WHO/HTM/TB/2007/287, Geneva: World Health Organization.

WHO (2008a) World Health Statistics 2008, Geneva: World Health Organization.

WHO (2008b) 'World Health Report calls for return to primary health care approach', WHO Media Centre, 14 October. http://www.who.int/mediacentre/news/releases/2008/pr38/en/index.html (accessed 1 November 2008).

WHO-WTO (2002) 'Differential Pricing and the Financing of Essential Drugs' in Granville, Brigitte (ed.) *The Economics of Essential Medicines*, London: Royal Institute of International Affairs, International Economics Programme.

World Trade Organization (WTO) (2001) *DOHA WTO Ministerial Declaration*, WT/MIN(01)/DEC/1, 20 November.

Wouters, Anne Marie (1991) 'Essential National Health Research in Developing Countries: Health Care Financing and the Quality of Care', *International Journal of Health Planning and Management*, 6, 253–271.

Yach, Derek and Douglas Bettcher (1998a) 'The Globalization of Public Health, I: Threats and Opportunities', *American Journal of Public Health*, 88(5), 735–738.

Yach, Derek and Douglas Bettcher (1998b) 'The Globalization of Public Health, II: The Convergence of Self-Interest and Altruism', *American Journal of Public Health*, 88(5), 738–741.

Yach, Derek, Heather Wipfli, Ross Hammond and Stanton Glantz (2007) 'Globalization and Tobacco', in Kawachi, Ichiro and Sarah Wamala (eds.) *Globalization and Health*, Oxford: Oxford University Press.

Yamin, Alicia Ely (1996) 'Defining Questions: Situating Issues of Power in the Formulation of a Right to Health under International Law', *Human Rights Quarterly*, 18(2), 398–438.

Yamin, Alicia Ely (2005) 'Learning to Dance: Bringing the Fields of Human Rights and Public Health Together to Promote Women's Well-Being', in Yamin, Alicia Ely (ed.), *Learning to Dance: Case Studies on Advancing Women's Reproductive Health and Well-Being from the Perspectives of Public Health and Human Rights*, Cambridge, Mass: Francois-Xavier Bagnoud Center Series on Health and Human Rights, Harvard University Press.

York, Anna (2002) 'Civilian Health: The New Target of Conflict', *Lancet*, 360, 1228.

Youde, Jeremy (2005) 'Enter the Fourth Horseman: Health Security and International Relations Theory', *Whitehead Journal of Diplomacy and International Relations*, 6(1), 193–208.

Zacher, Mark W. (2007) 'The Transformation in Global Health Collaboration since the 1990s', in Cooper, Andrew F., John J. Kirton and Ted Schrecker (eds.) *Governing Global Health: Challenge, Response, Innovation*, Aldershot: Ashgate.

Zwi, Anthony B. and Fatima Alvarez-Castillo (2003) 'Forced Migration, Globalisation, and Public Health: Getting the Big Picture into Focus', in Allotey, Pascale (ed.) *The Health of Refugees: Public Health Perspectives from Crisis to Settlement*, Melbourne: Oxford University Press.

INDEX